AF575243

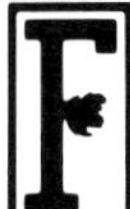

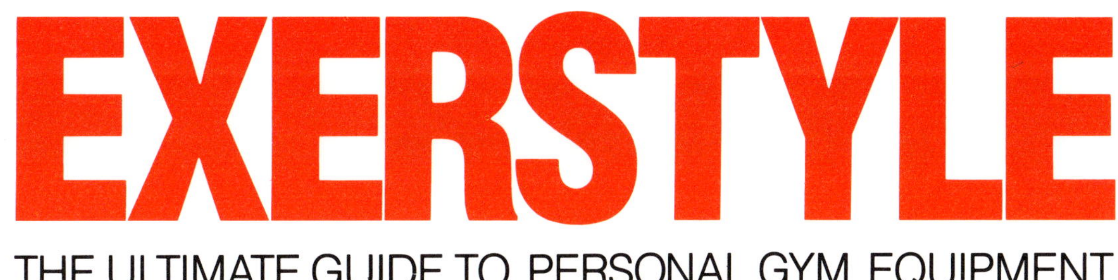

PHILIP MAZZURCO

A FIRESIDE BOOK
Published by
Simon and Schuster
New York

A QUARTO BOOK

Published by Simon and Schuster
A Division of Simon & Schuster, Inc.
Rockefeller Center
1230 Avenue of the Americas
New York, New York 10020

Library of Congress Cataloging in Publication Data
Main entry under title:

Exerstyle: the ultimate guide to personal gym equipment.

"Fireside book."
1. Gymnasiums—Apparatus and equipment. 2. Physical fitness—Equipment and supplies.
GV409.E94 1985 796.4′06′8028 85-2124
ISBN 0-671-55204-X

EXERSTYLE: The Ultimate Guide to Personal Gym Equipment
was prepared and produced by
Quarto Marketing Ltd.
15 West 26th Street
New York, New York 10010

Art Director: Richard Boddy
Designer: Rod Gonzalez
Photo Research: Susan M. Duane
Editorial Assistant: Louise Quayle
Illustrations: Louis Pappas

Typeset by BPE Graphics, Inc.
Color separations by Hong Kong Scanner Craft Company Ltd.
Printed and bound in Hong Kong by Leefung-Asco Printers Ltd.

• DEDICATION •

For John
Whose advice
and insights
establish
a standard
against which
to measure
my own.

ACKNOWLEDGMENTS

For • ROBERT FERKEL, upon whose friendship I've come to rely for the depth of his personal and professional understanding; • RUBÉN DE SAAVEDRA, whose considerable knowledge and provocative insights are enlivened with great charm, warmth, and sincerity; • ROGER GROSS, who expedites my project requests with seldom-encountered wit, humor, and spirit; • KATHERINE STEPHENS, who unselfishly encourages my work and strengthens my confidence at every opportunity; • LILLI LIHN, to whom I owe a debt of gratitude for professional efforts on my behalf; • JAMES FRANKLIN MITCHELL, whose unsolicited help on this book and shared professional contacts have proven to be invaluable assets; • ERIC BERNARD, who unselfishly offers his work and thoughtful cooperation regarding my editorial endeavors; • BOB PATINO and • VINCENT WOLF, who so readily share their work as well as professional advice and leads; • MICHAEL MATINZI, whose charm, polish, and flawless professionalism redefine the consummate publicist; • MARIO BUATTA, a belated thank-you for his help on *The Media Design Book;* • CLAIRE SHELLEY, whose unpretentious, matter-of-fact approach to my photo requests is relieved by her ribald sense of humor and sharp wit; • KATHRYN PAIGE, whose kindness and warmth makes doing business with her a rare pleasure; all the designers, architects, and photographers, especially • PHILLIP ENNIS, who beautifully documented my locations, without whom these books would not be possible; • ROY JUDA, who invaluably assisted at the equipment photographing session; • T.C., who is and shall always be T.L.O.M.L. A very special thank you to my editor, • MARTA HALLETT, whose balanced professionalism and sense of humor created an encouraging climate in which to write.

CONTENTS

CONTENTS

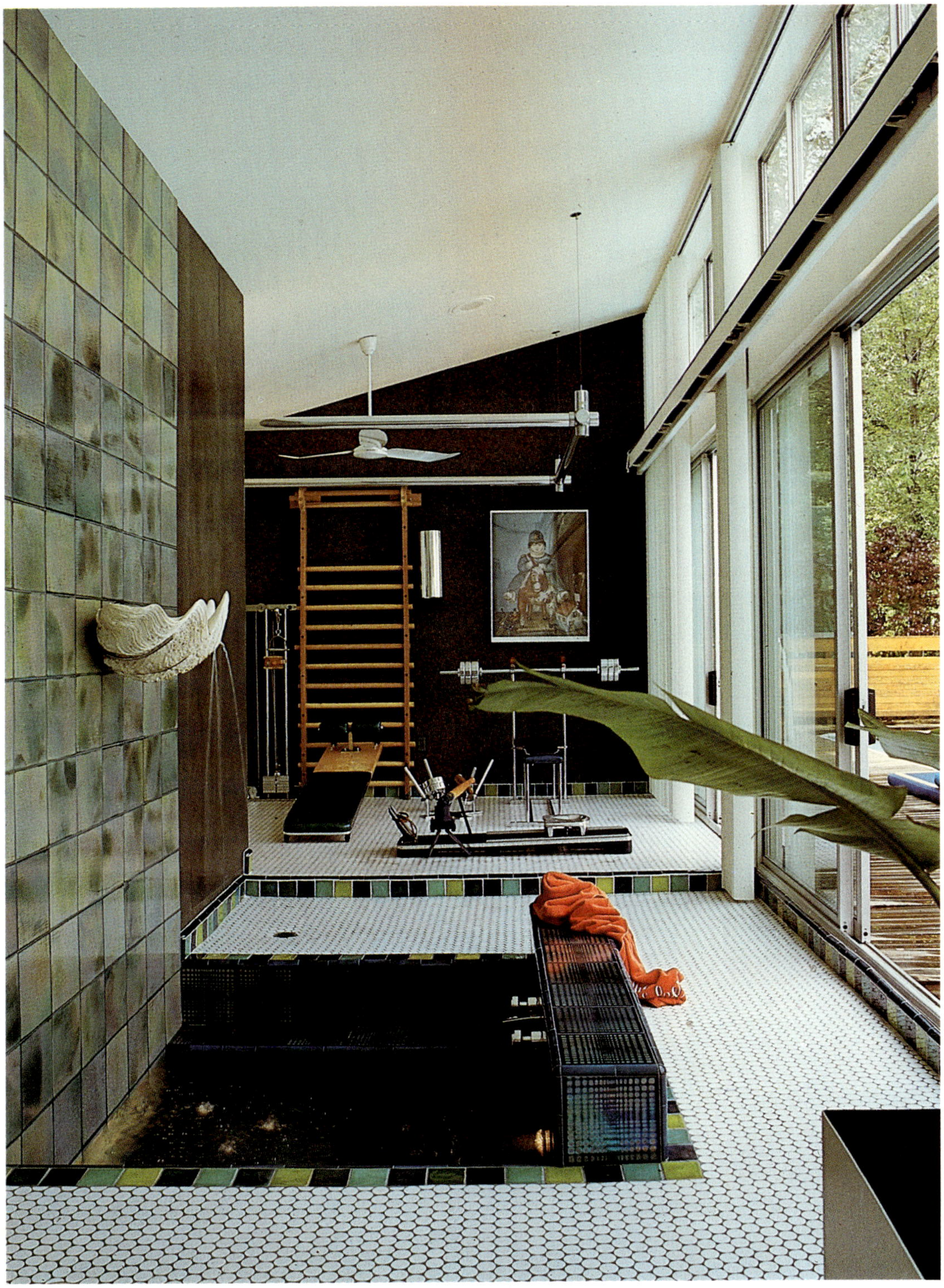

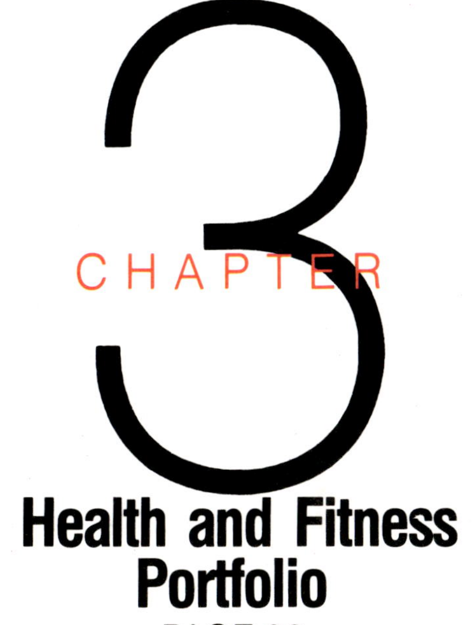

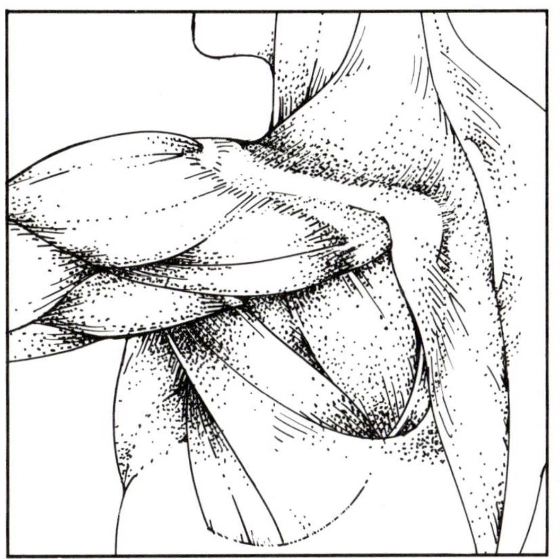

INTRODUCTION

WORKING OUT AT HOME

Working out in the comfort of the home has recently become a popular option for more and more people who are fitness-minded. Home gymnasiums are springing up in basements, spare rooms, apartment alcoves, and anywhere else that fitness paraphernalia can be utilized. Riding the crest of this trend is a whole new generation of exercise apparatuses—a staggering array of advanced, ingenious, and compact systems, each with a variety of fitness capabilities. At one time the stay-at-home exerciser had almost no alternative but to take a solitary spin on a trusty stationary bicycle. No longer: Today's home-fitness enthusiast can also row, bench press, and run, on high-tech equipment that may be the envy of many a health club.

As the home gym threatens to displace the gourmet kitchen or luxurious bath as the chief status symbol, physical fitness has become big business. Personal gymnasium gear has mushroomed into a $500 million a year business that's expected to double within the next four years. Recognizing the vast market potential, many of the commercial manufacturers have introduced home lines or expanded already-existing ones, while new companies continue to flood the market with ingenious products and an unforseen competitive spirit that is challenging commercial clubs.

Until about five years ago, few people could afford the luxury of bringing the health club into the home. Most major exercise equipment was designed for commercial use both in size and price. In recent years, however, the home market has muscled in on the health club territory with the introduction of bodybuilding instruments that are portable, affordable, and well-designed. In addition to weight training machines, there are folding bicycles for pedaling in place, compact rowing machines, electronically driven treadmills, and even recirculating staircases. Today new developments have even applied technology to classic exercise equipment in the form of microprocessors, which can monitor everything from heartbeat to caloric expenditure.

Even though many people are motivated by the group dynamics of health clubs, several factors have drawn consumers back home to shape up. The first is time. The continuing fitness obsession has filled most health clubs to capacity, and waiting on line to use a piece of equipment is something we can all do without. Working out at home also allows you the luxury of scheduling exercise at your own convenience rather than in conjunction with a health club's hours. Comfort is another factor. More often than not, a beginner will prefer to go through the awkward learning stages without an audience. Mothers with preschool children find working out at home more convenient than finding a babysitter. And, of course, there are those who consider working out at home to be more cost efficient in view of the spiraling membership fees of the health clubs.

Before going out to buy equipment for a home gym, there are some basic considerations to examine. The critical first step is determining the appropriate equipment. What is appropriate depends on your age, sex, goals, and current fitness level, and is best determined with the help of a physician and health-care professional. Space and budget are the next considerations. While any area of a house or apartment can accommodate a home gym, a basement is ideal for weight work. The sound of weights being lowered to the floor or crashing to the bottom of a stack on a stationary unit in the upper rooms of a house can reverberate throughout the house. This is even worse in an apartment with a downstairs neighbor.

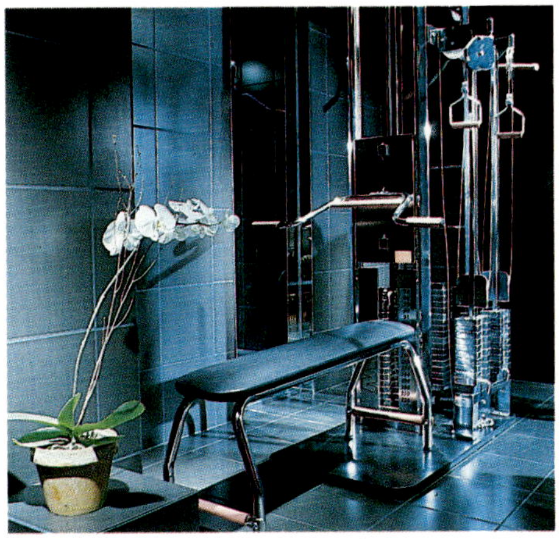

But whatever area is chosen, it should be carpeted to muffle sound as well as to reduce impact on feet, especially if you will be running in place or jumping rope. Good lighting and adequate ventilation are also important for obvious reasons. Mirrors are helpful to check one's form while performing a routine or working with free weights. Television can help distract one from the monotony of cycling or stationary running. Music also helps as a distraction and it sets the mood and pace.

Exercise is ultimately a personal activity. Before determining which kind of exercise is best, you must determine what you want to achieve. Adults are usually concerned with maintaining strength and stamina, avoiding increases in body weight and fat, and avoiding potential health problems that occur with a sedentary lifestyle. Others exercise for cosmetic reasons, such as figure control, or even psychological ones. But whatever the reason, exercise can preserve and enhance the quality of your life by increasing your physical capability for work and play. A properly conceived exercise program provides the individual with an all-around feeling of well-being and a healthy, well-conditioned body.

Whether the goal is weight loss, muscle tone, or cardiovascular conditioning, exercise promotes physical fitness. Fitness is particularly important for the heart, for when the heart is properly exercised, it pumps blood more efficiently, keeping all parts of the body properly oxygenated. Scientists are now convinced that proper exercise leading to an increase in endurance fitness is a significant factor in reducing the severity of cardiovascular and other diseases.

Aerobic exercises are most often recommended in fitness programs because they are primarily designed for cardiovascular conditioning. Aerobic means in the presence of oxygen. Aerobic exercises are continuous physical activity that utilize the large muscles for an extended period of time, thereby stimulating the circulatory system to increase the blood flow throughout the body. An exchange mechanism is created whereby the blood oxygenates and replaces the waste products in the muscles.

Examples of aerobic exercises are cycling, rowing, walking, jogging, swimming, and jumping rope. Aerobic exercises like these are *isotonic*—they incorporate rhythmic, repetitive motion in which large muscles are stretched repeatedly. Sports activities such as tennis, soccer, and basketball are referred to as *anaerobic* (without oxygen) exercises. These are characterized by stop-and-go activity in which specific small muscle groups are exercised in short bursts of energy. Anaerobic exercise is not conducive to cardiovascular conditioning because at each stop the heart rate slows down, then has to be restarted. While this kind of exercise certainly benefits the cardiovascular system, it should augment regular conditioning programs.

Another beneficial kind of exercise is *isometric*, in which muscles are exercised in resistance to weight. Here specific muscles are involved, and the benefit to the cardiovascular system is minimal. Weightlifting is a good example of this kind of exercise. Weightlifting does, however, promote muscular strength, definition, and tone. It also provides many of the psychological benefits attributable to fitness training, especially a general sense of well-being and self-esteem.

Physical fitness is a way of life; one that requires lifetime dedication in order for there to be continuous reinforcement of its benefits. Your program should, most of all, be rewarding. Consider your specific goals as well as your social inclinations. The kind of exercise that is best for you, then, is that which allows you to achieve your goals in a pleasant manner so that you will want to continue to exercise regularly.

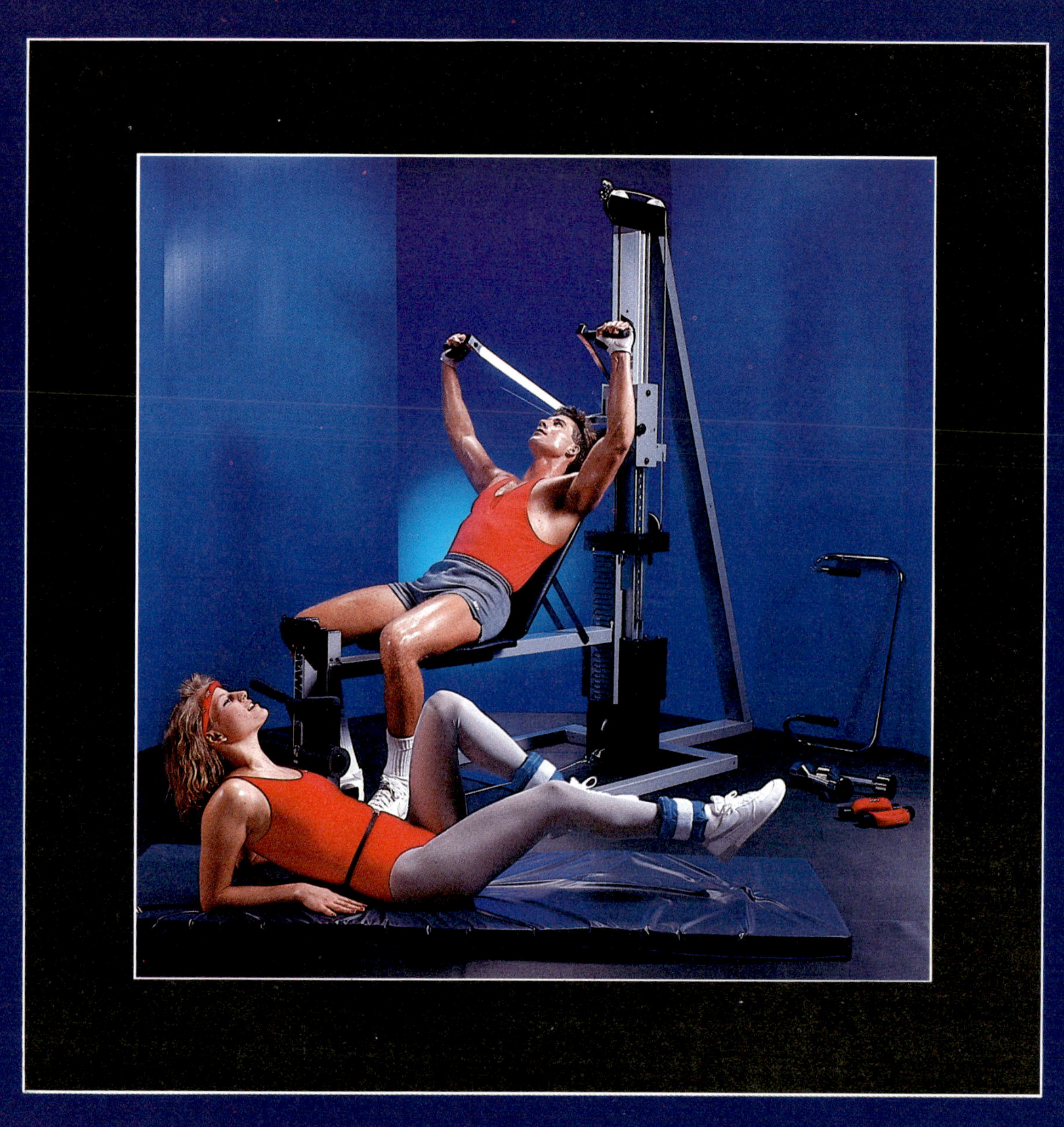

CHAPTER
ONE

EQUIPMENT PORTFOLIO

A whole new generation of exercise apparatus has emerged for scores of people who are now coming home to exercise. Until about five years ago, however, few people could afford to bring the luxuries of the health club home with them. Most major exercise equipment was designed for commercial use, both in terms of size and price. But in the last five years things have changed. The new home fitness market has generated a variety of attractively designed and sensibly scaled equipment especially for home use. Even the latest electronic advances have been incorporated into such tune-up gadgets as vital signs monitors, pulsimeters, and pedometers.

Before selecting any home equipment, the first thing to decide is, what kind of exercise you want to do. Once the activity has been determined you will want to consider the amount of time to be invested in an effective program and, of course, spatial accommodations. And naturally, cost will be a factor, too. Since physical fitness requires lifetime dedication, the quality and endurance of the equipment must be a major consideration. You will, after all, want to achieve your fitness goals in an enjoyable manner and in an environment which will encourage you to exercise regularly.

This chapter will help you through the dizzying array of equipment currently available. It presents a full picture on selected home pieces from all the major equipment groups. Brief introductions outline the general benefits of the equipment category and then discuss the design, construction, and use of the individual models. In selecting equipment for inclusion, the cost, size, utility, and efficiency have been evaluated. Each group introduction specifically outlines the criteria for the particular type of equipment.

The chapter is organized by equipment type. Whether you want a multipurpose gym or merely one devoted to performance of a single type of exercise, it is crucial to select the right equipment. Beginning with cardiovascular conditioning, the chapter includes muscular conditioning, inversion therapy, general equipment, and accessories, running the gamut from stationary bicycles, rowing machines, treadmills, and trampolines to recirculating stairs and home saunas.

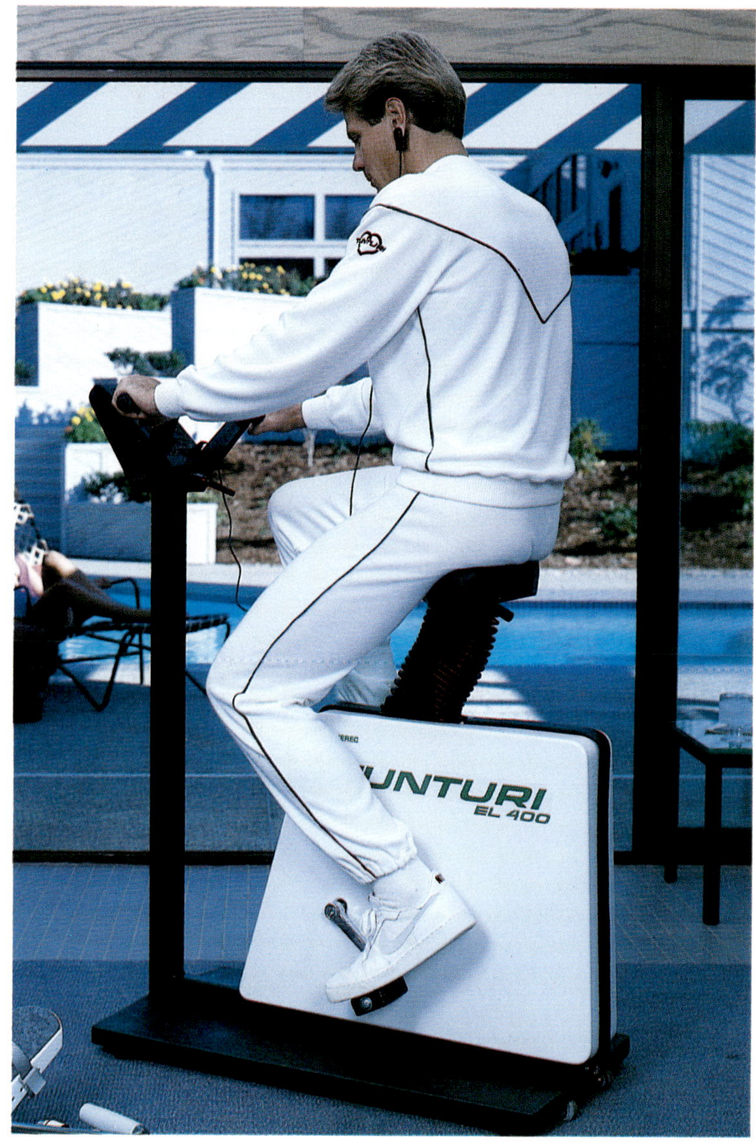

STATIONARY BICYCLES

Stationary bicycles are probably the best machines for a cardiovascular conditioning program. In selecting one, look for a solid frame that is able to support you without untoward movement of the machine. A heavy frame and a solid flywheel are the most important features of a good bicycle. The flywheel helps set the resistance; it should rotate smoothly when you are pedaling. A solid flywheel—usually cast iron is best—will also tend to resist warping from the heat generated by the activity. With this type of cardiovascular conditioning program, it is important that the exercise be easily and exactly replicated each time it is performed. As your body becomes acclimated to one resistance, you should systematically increase the resistance you use. This process of requiring more effort by increasing the resistance is called *progressive resistance.* It requires an exercise machine that allows progressive and accurate adjustment of resistance. Those bicycles that can quantitatively measure effort, can allow exercises to be precisely replicated, and increase the challenge in accurate increments are called ergometers. They are the best stationary bicycles available.

A recommended type of workout for the exercise bicycle alternates intervals of work with intervals of rest or light exercise. Called interval training, it has been used by athletes for many years and has been extremely successful in improving endurance, or heart-lung fitness. While the relief interval should generally consist of some type of activity, it is the work interval that demands more attention. The four important aspects of the work interval are: (1) the distance covered (miles); (2) the time taken to cover the distance; (3) the speed of the ride (mph); and (4) the heart rate during the rides. On some bikes these parameters are automatically monitored and displayed on a readout generally located at the handlebars.

Precor 830e Bicycle Ergometer

The Precor 830e Bicycle Ergometer features high-tech styling and precision craftsmanship. The sturdy but slender frame is constructed with strong anodized aircraft aluminum and finished in either brushed silver and matte black. A low step-in height facilitates mounting and dismounting, while the horizontal flywheel provides a very stable base. Completely sealed bearings with direct drive never need lubricating, making the 830e virtually maintenance-free. A battery-powered microprocessor mounted between the handlebars provides elapsed time, pedaling rpm, distance, and caloric expenditure. A wide contoured foam seat with locking increments is adjustable in height, while the cushioned handlebar grips are adjustable through 360° of articulation.

Located between the handlebars, the microprocessor monitors crucial pulse data and is powered by an easily replaceable 9-volt alkaline battery.

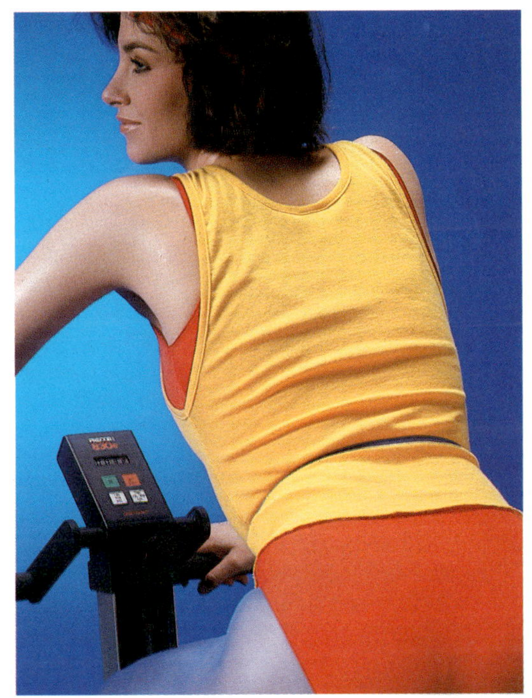

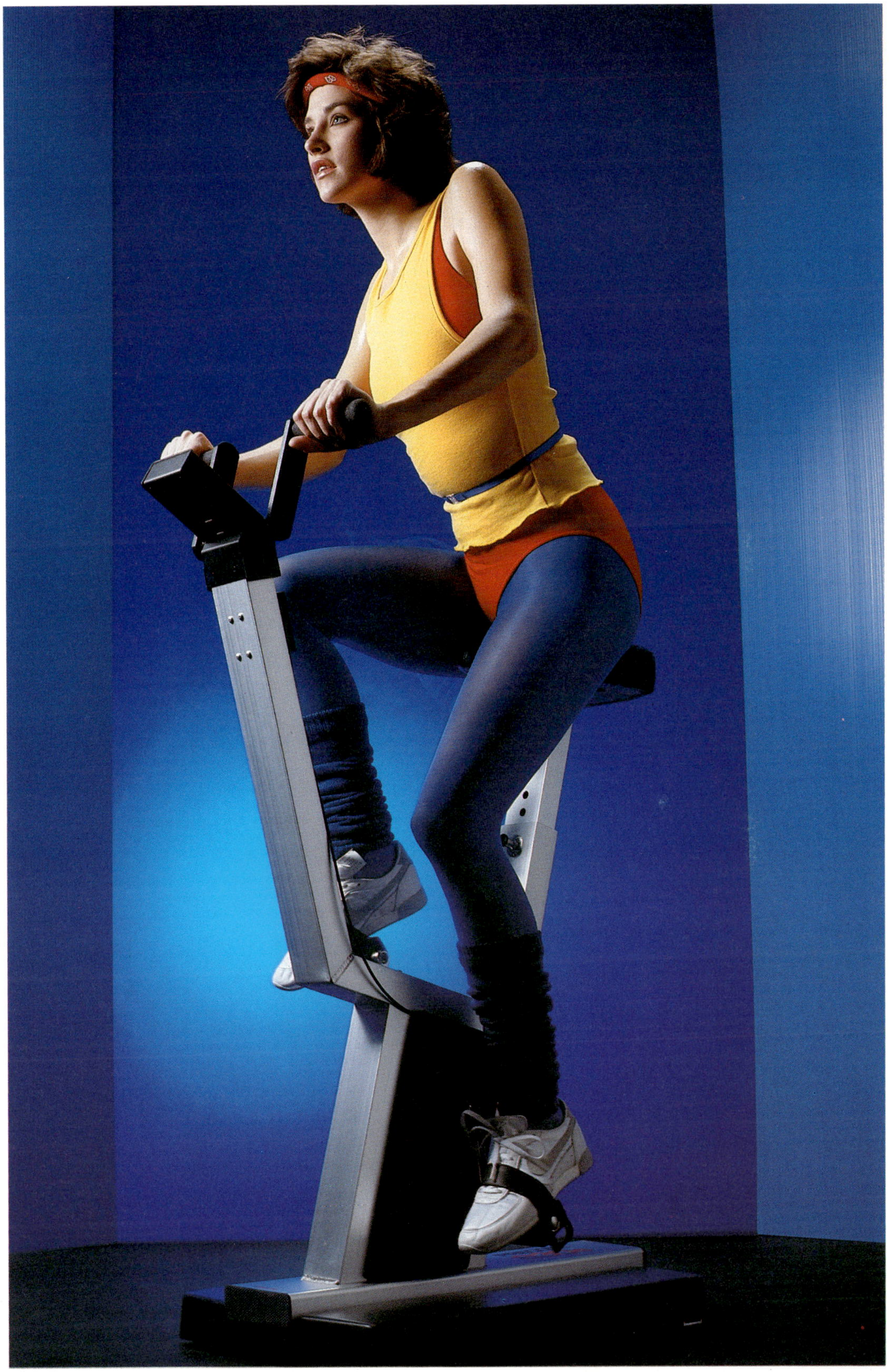

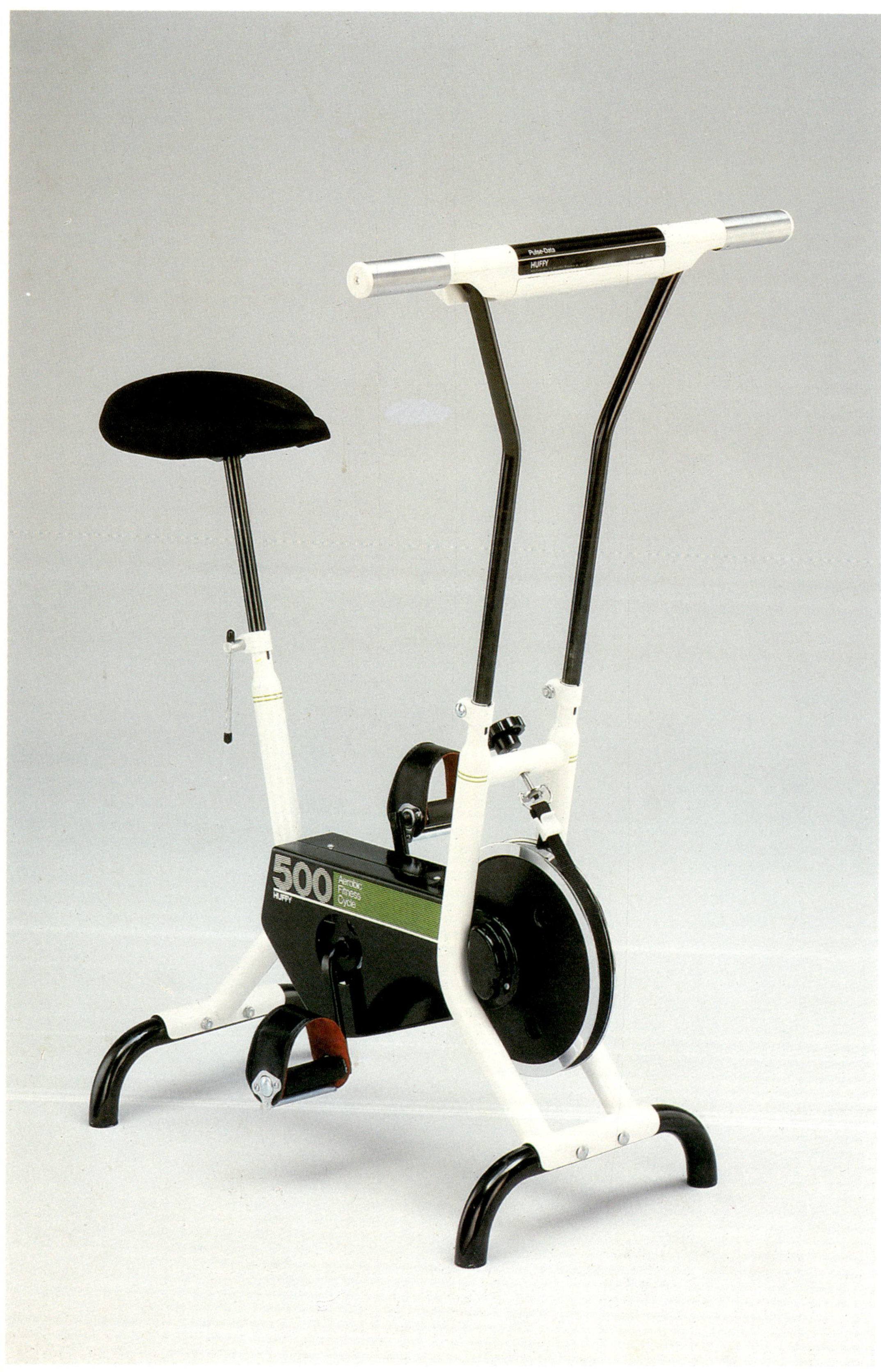

The Pulse Data unit is horizontally mounted between the handlebars for a dashboard-like effect.

Huffy Aerobic Fitness 500 Cycle Model 90953

Huffy's Aerobic Fitness 500 Cycle Model 90953 is a high-styled compact bike featuring a heavy-duty steel, step-through H-frame. Finished in Arctic White, the bike features a solid chrome, cast flywheel and an easy-to-operate belt tension system. The dashboard-style Pulse Data console, mounted between the handlebars, shows elapsed time, pulse rate, distance traveled, and miles per hour. The deluxe contoured saddle features a quick-adjust mechanism, while the dual handlebars are also adjustable. Wide stabilizer bars and a fully enclosed chain guard assure safe, quiet operation.

Monarch Mark II

The Monarch Mark II is actually a more refined version of Monarch's Mark I. The tubular steel welded frame is finished in white baked enamel with blue accents. A double chain guard and built-in drive exchange give the Mark II a neat, unfussy appearance. Specially designed Monarch handlebars feature a unique configuration that allow for as many as six different grip positions. The single handlebar can also be turned and therefore changed directionally. A completely solid flywheel assures a smooth ride, while resistance is controlled by an adjustable control knob. A three-gauge instrument panel is mounted atop the chain guard: The wattmeter shows energy output measured in watts; the speedometer shows speed of the wheel and distance traveled; and also included is a timer to measure elapsed time. The Monarch Mark II also offers a choice of two saddles, wide and extra wide. Both are adjustable by a nonslip, quick-lock mechanism.

The EL-400 control panel with built-in pulsimeter, stopwatch, metronome, pedaling speed monitor, and workload setting. The entire panel can pivot 360° for added convenience.

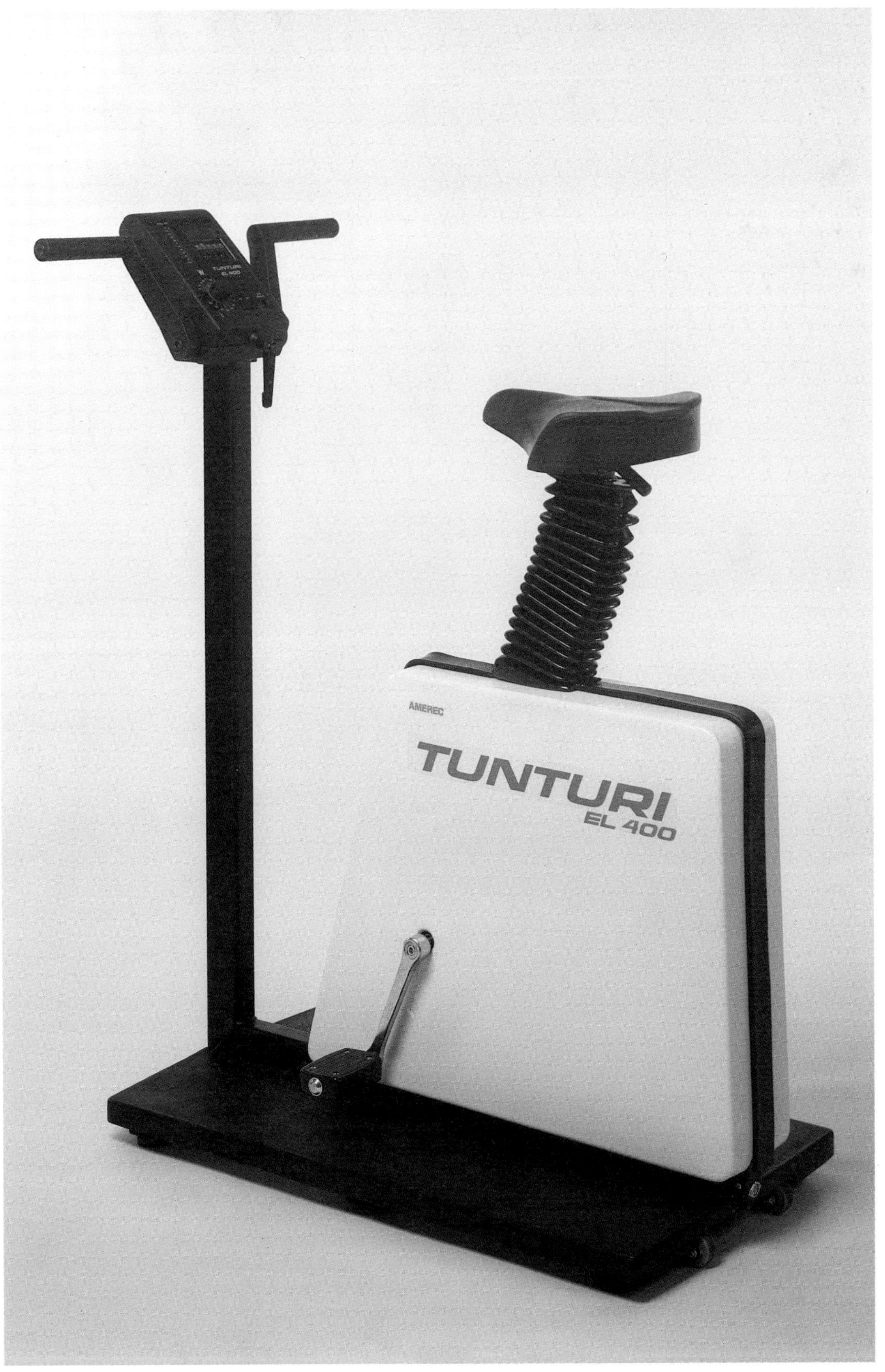

Tunturi EL 400 Electronic Ergometer

The Tunturi EL 400 Electronic Ergometer combines futuristic styling with advanced electronics. Both the electronically controlled pedaling mechanism and saddle are encased in a slim, baked-enamel housing, while the matte black handlebars and pulse data unit are supported by a tubular steel upright. The EL 400 was conceived to eliminate the possible sources of error in obtaining test results. The pedaling mechanism, for example, is totally regulated by an electronically controlled circulating current brake; pedaling efficiency is therefore automatically regulated. A pulsimeter with LED (Light Emitting Diode) readouts is mounted between the handlebars. By attaching the ear sensor to the earlobe, the pulsimeter's 4-bit microcomputer will process heartbeats into pulse readouts. The control panel also incorporates a stopwatch, pedaling speed indicator, pedaling speed efficiency control indicator setting, and a convenient metronome to set a program pace. Both the anatomically formed cushion seat and handlebars are adjustable.

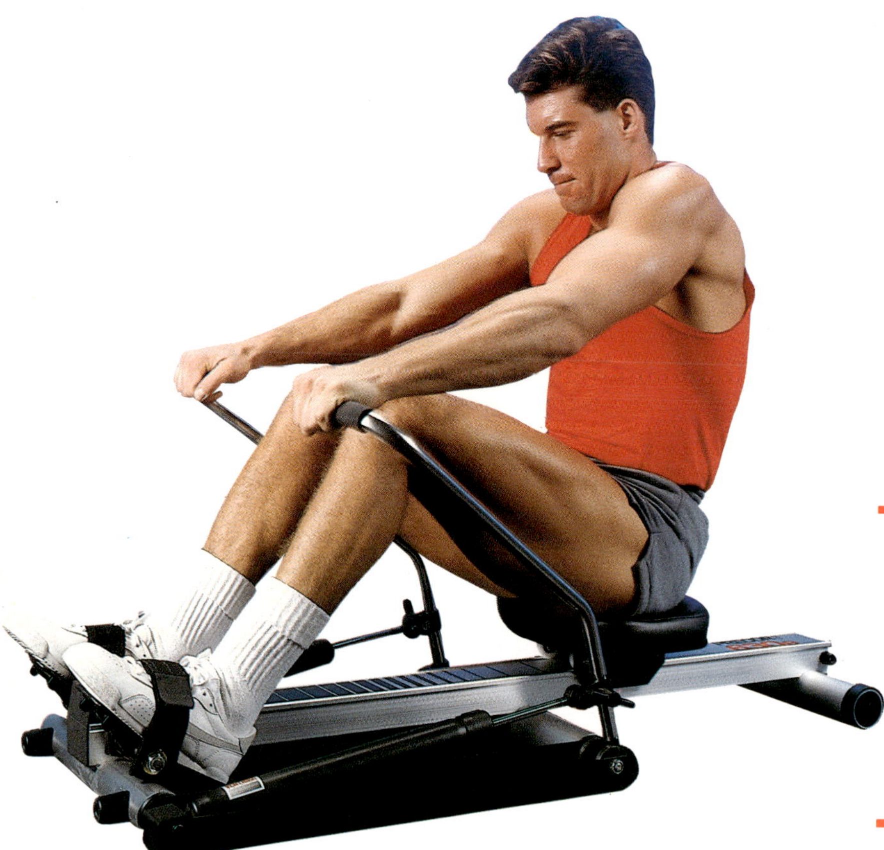

ROWING MACHINES

Rowing is one of the most beneficial exercises, because it provides a total body workout in one continuous action. Rowing machines—perhaps the most complicated of the home devices for cardiovascular conditioning—are combination units providing both aerobic and anaerobic exercise, increasing respiratory and cardiovascular fitness while developing all major muscle groups, including back, stomach, arms, shoulders, and legs. The machine can also help develop special muscle groups—with special exercises such as arm pulls, deltoid/tricep pulls, squats, and sit-ups.

The unique rhythmic action of the rowing exercise also strengthens the heart and circulatory system, elevating the heartbeat to 80% of its potential maximum. Rowing machines will definitely suit your needs if muscle conditioning is as important to you as is good cardiovascular fitness and health.

Initially, however, using the machine will not immediately benefit both systems—in most people. The musculature is generally weaker than the cardiovascular system and so a longer time must be spent exercising on rowers in order to achieve cardiovascular benefit. In other words, the weaker musculature system is unable to generate enough vigor initially to build the heart rate to the target zone: Exercising on the rowing machine will benefit the muscles rather than the heart. Ultimately, the musculature will catch up to the development level of the cardiovascular system, at which point workouts begin to benefit both systems.

When selecting a rowing machine, look for one with an adequately weighted frame to keep the rower in place even during the most strenuous workouts. Resistance pistons should be sealed and constructed of heavy-gauge metal; the contoured seat should ride smoothly and quietly over the monorail.

Additional features to look for are: seat padding, back support, comfortable handgrips, convenient footstraps, and wheels or castors, which will facilitate both easy storage and movement.

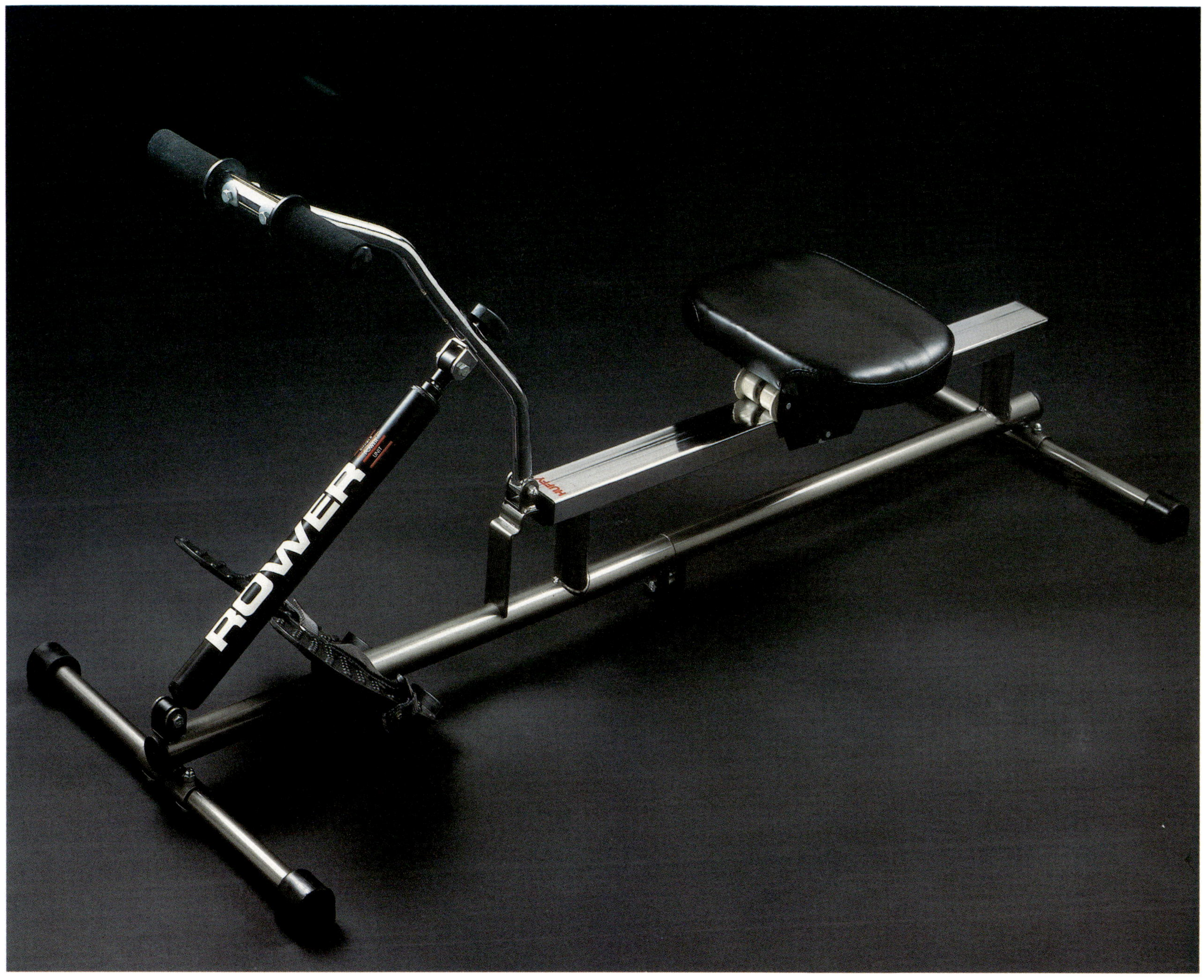

The Huffy 6995 Aerobic Rowing System features a single actuating hydraulic piston with three adjustable tension positions. The 6995's box beam and tube construction is finished in metallic gray.

Huffy 6995 Aerobic Rowing System

The Huffy 6995 Aerobic Rowing System features the popular high-tech look with metallic gray and black frame and accents. Rather than dual-piston resistance, the 6995 uses a single actuating hydraulic piston, which is adjustable to three tension positions. A single handlebar attached to the piston has comfortable black foam grips. The black, contoured padded seat glides along a box beam monorail; while the rest of the frame is of tubular construction. Wide stabilizer bars ensure smooth operation and are fitted with nonskid rubber tips. Molded black foot pedals have fastening straps for added security.

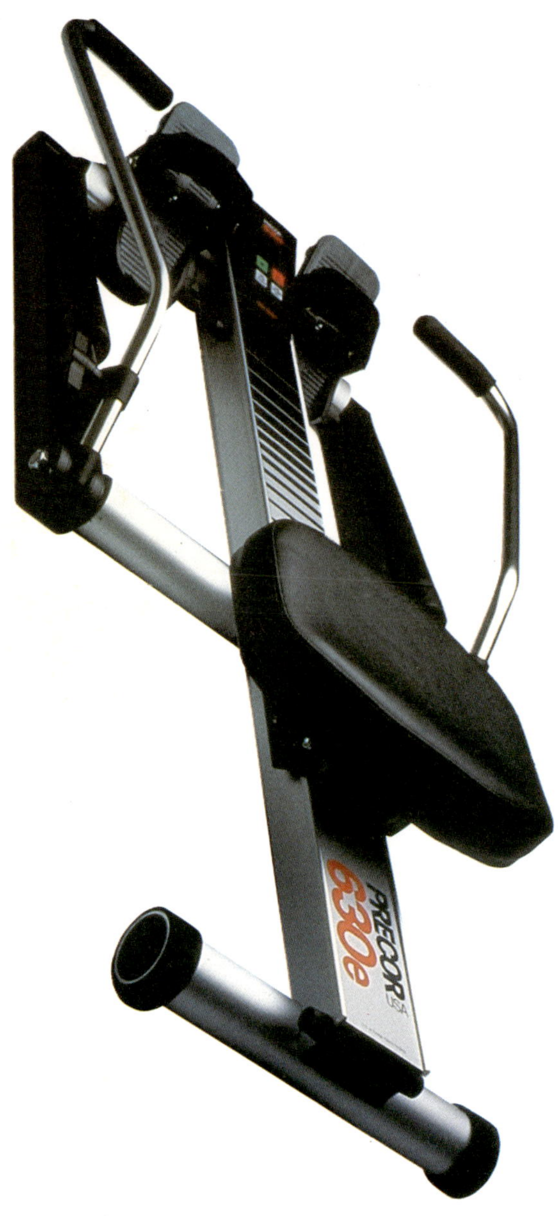

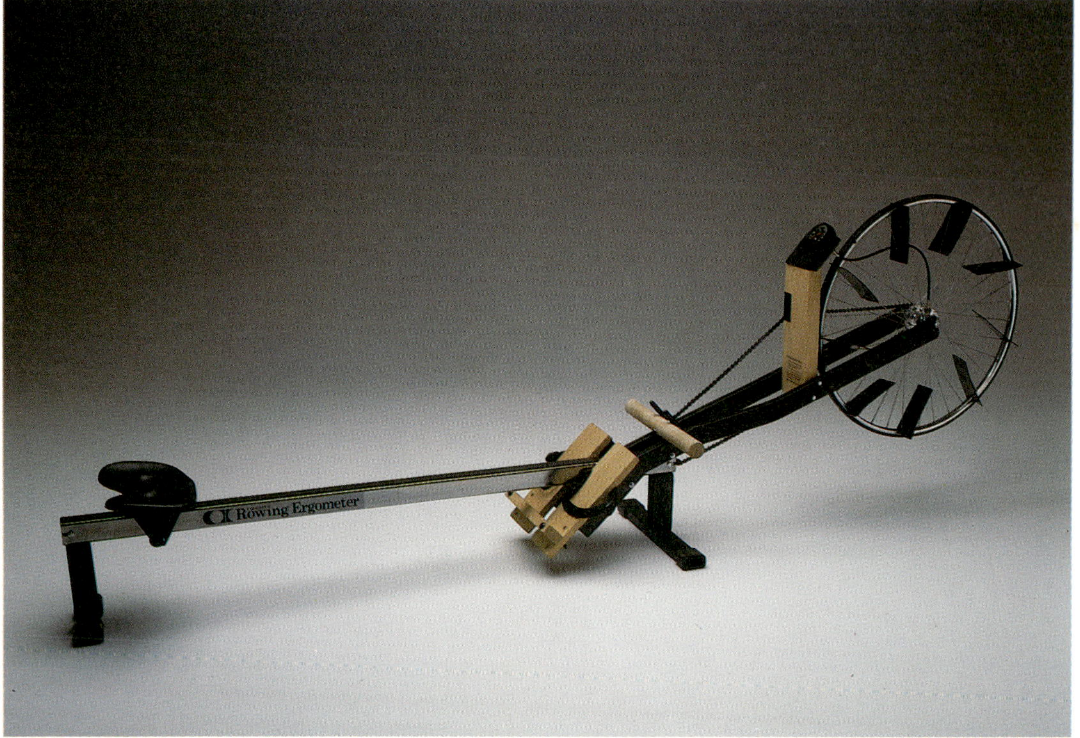

Scullers Ergometer

Despite its almost outmoded design profile (the machine seems to sacrifice for precision and accuracy), the Scullers Ergometer is billed as the only exercise rowing machine designed to simulate actual rowing conditions. The chrome-plated heavy-gauge steel and hardwood frame supports a precision-geared direct-drive chain mechanism and open-spoked flywheel with plastic wind blades. Rotating the flywheel creates air resistance that simulates the actual water drag on the hull of a boat. Since the flywheel builds momentum with each stroke, the rower feels a sense of acceleration just as if he were increasing speed in the water. The resistance level can be easily controlled by engaging various-sized drive-chain sprockets, while a speedometer and odometer permit careful monitoring of expended energy. A contoured seat glides on the chrome-plated monorail and features sealed ball-bearing rollers, which never need lubricating. The machine also features nylon straps to hold feet in place and nonskid rubber feet. The entire frame folds for easy storage.

Located between the footpads is a sealed microprocessor that displays such information as elapsed time and caloric expenditure. It is powered by an easily replaceable 9-volt alkaline battery.

Precor 630e Rowing Ergometer

The Precor 630e Rowing Ergometer has a brushed aluminum frame accented with black—giving a decidedly sleek design. For strength and maneuverability, the frame's material is anodized aircraft aluminum; the rowing arms are polished chrome/stainless steel with black padded handgrips. Dual oil-filled resistance pistons ensure smooth and consistent strokes. A comfortably contoured seat slides smoothly on a full ball-bearing seat carriage system. Because the frame is larger than those of standard models, it can accommodate any size of user. Fully rotating foot pedals feature adjustable Velcro straps to hold the feet securely in place. Located between the footpads is a sealed microprocessor-controlled electronics unit that displays elapsed time, total strokes, work rate in calories per minute during the exercise period, and total caloric expenditure. The entire machine is stored easily in an upright position.

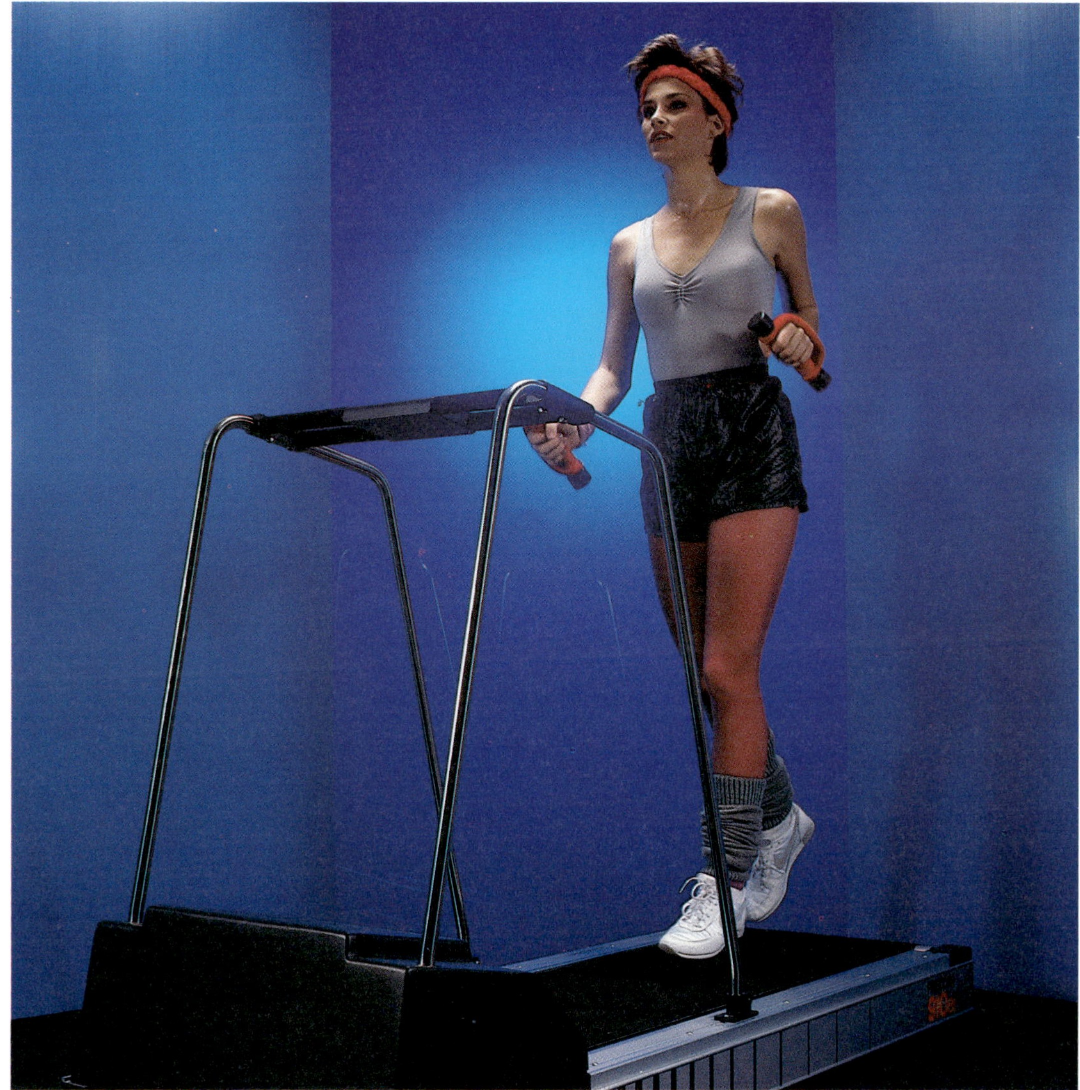

The microprocessor-based sealed control features easy-to-read LED display and pressure-sensitive controls.

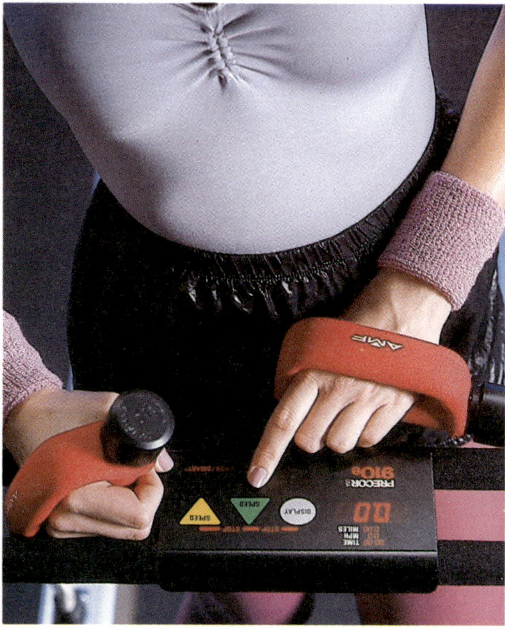

TREADMILLS

Treadmills replicate walking, jogging, or running exercises and therefore are another way to achieve cardiovascular conditioning. The most basic treadmills are manual and are used for walking or running at a pace set by the user. Electronic treadmills, on the other hand, enable you to establish a running speed that must be maintained, thus preventing you from periodically easing up on the exercise when you begin to tire.

When selecting a home treadmill, look for solidly built models with stable handrails. The machine should also be wide enough so that it doesn't wobble even when inclined. Better machines will come equipped with fingertip control panels for accurate measurement of your progress, as well as a running bed incline adjustment to enhance difficulty.

Precor 910ei

An anodized aluminum frame and black accents reinforce the high-tech image of Precor's 910ei treadmill. A specially regulated motor prevents momentary surges or stalls from your footplant. A fingertip key pad puts you on your predetermined pace from one mph to eight mph, adjustable to the tenth of a mile. Rather than an odometer, the 910ei uses a light strobe, which is more accurate and sensitive, to measure speed and distance.

Cushioned handgrips bridge the gap between the tubular handrails and hold a digital display unit. Total elapsed time, speed, and total mileage can all be shown; press the display switch and you can alternately monitor time, distance, and speed at 5-second intervals. The 910ei running surface is an antistatic, nonstretch elastomer belt over a slider surface.

The 910ei also has a gas-assisted spring arm (more for convenience than anything) which inclines the running bed to simulate hills. The inclinometer gives you a precise measurement of the inclined elevation from 0 to 15% grade.

A microprocessor controlled 16-digit LED display panel is situated between the safety handles. Percent of grade, distance, time, speed, and pace can be accurately set and recorded. Readouts and machine speed automatically return to zero when machine is turned off.

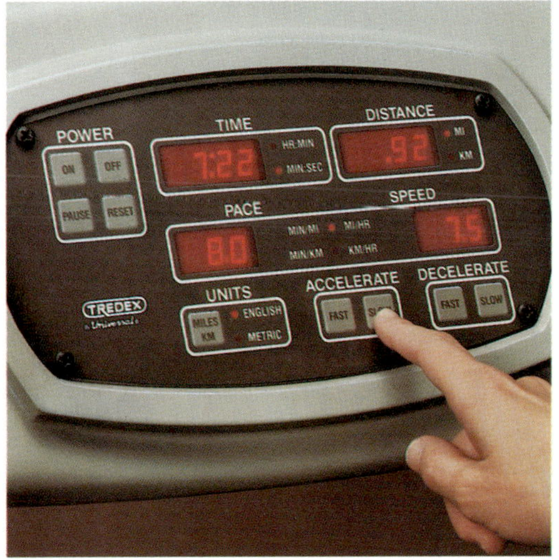

Tredex 2904

The Tredex 2904 treadmill features a futuristic look with an S-curved housing fabricated in NORYL structural foam (with a soil-resistant coating). It is powered by a direct-drive DC motor electronically controlled to provide infinitely varied speeds. The running bed is a brown elastomer belt on a no-stretch polyester backing that travels across a silicone-treated birchwood surface for comfortable running. Tubular molded safety handles provide stability when starting or stopping and serve as emergency shutoff when pushed downward. The black glass control panel is flushmounted between the handles and allows fingertip on-off and speed control. It shows speed, time, distance, and pulse rate in bright LED digits. The pulse rate sensor is mounted in a lightweight, adjustable belt, comes with reusable/disposable electrodes, and plugs directly into the control panel.

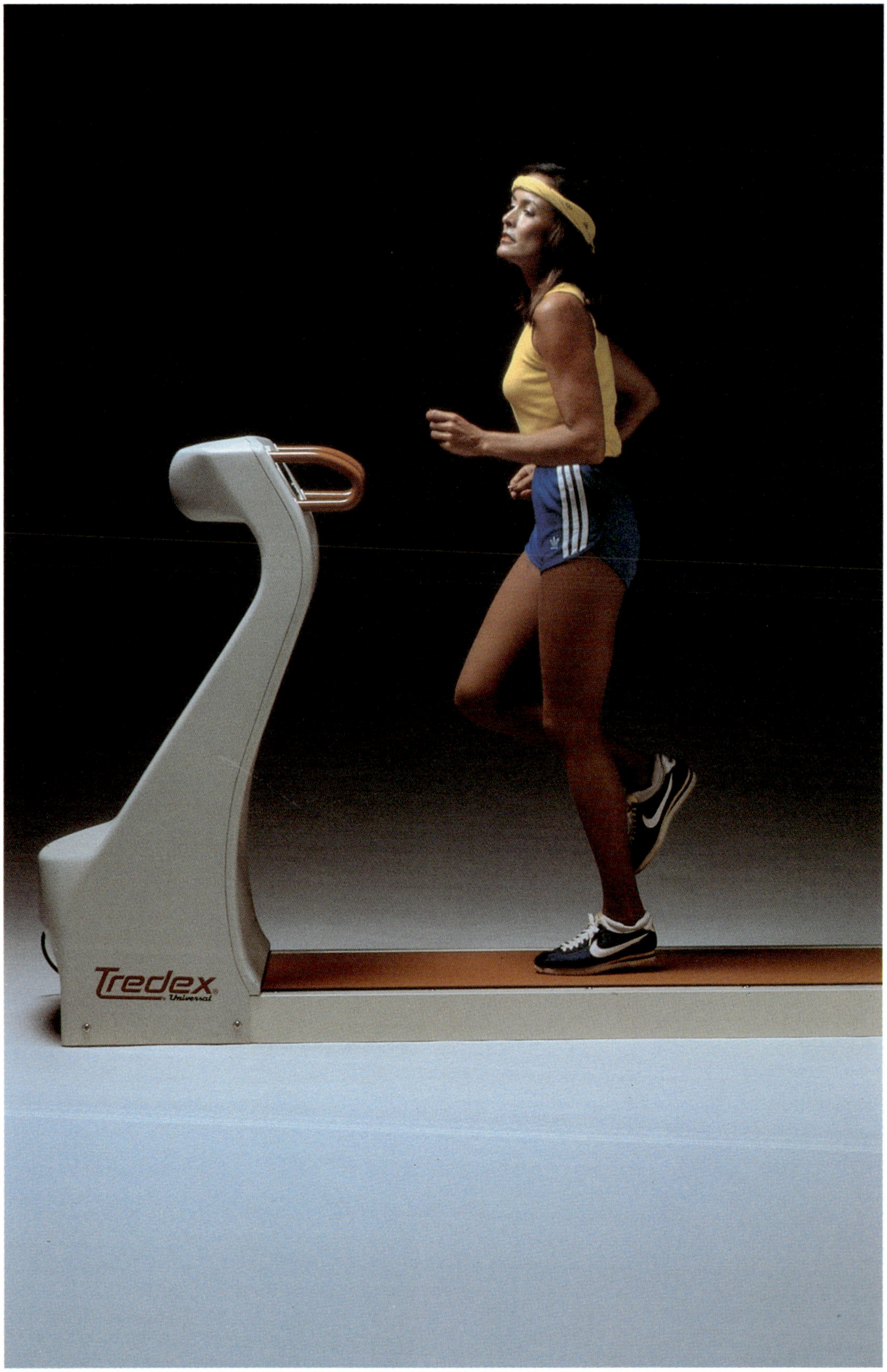

TRAMPOLINES

Rebound exercise platforms (trampolines) are best utilized as an alternate part of a vigorous jogging program. Although jogging and running are efficient exercises, the continuous pounding of the feet on hard surfaces can cause damage to the bones, joints, and tendons. Rebound exercise is therefore recommended because it offers protection to the weight-bearing joints. The platform's flexible, shock-absorbing surface is easy on the feet, ankles, and legs, allowing you to run, jog, or dance in place in total comfort. It has been shown, in fact, that a regimen of cushioned aerobics can relieve stress on the weight-bearing joints by as much as 85%. Increased balance, coordination, and timing are additional benefits of rebound exercise. And lastly, from a convenience standpoint, rebound exercise platforms permit continuity of your fitness program at home unhampered by inclement weather, traffic, or uneven terrain, as with the other home exercise equipment discussed. All the designs are the same. Limitations arise only when lesser-grade materials are used.

When selecting a home rebounder, look for a heavy-gauge steel frame double-welded for added strength. Springs should be made of galvanized steel to adequately support a durable polypropylene rebounding surface. There should also be a thick safety frame pad running along the entire circumference of the platform.

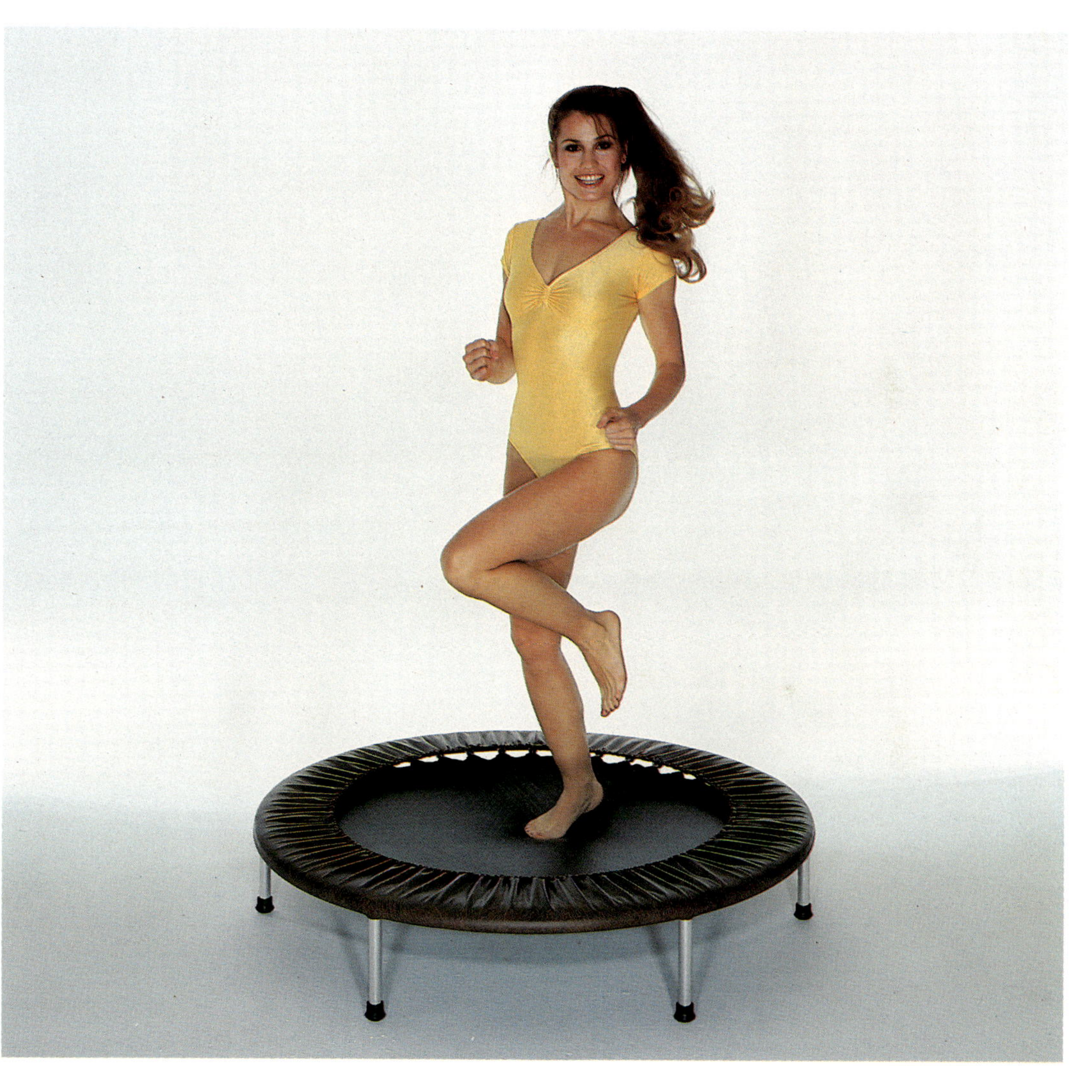

AMF Round Rebound Exerciser 470-008

This AMF 38-inch Round Rebounder is easy on the legs and offers better bounce because it offers 7/8-inch-diameter steel springs as anchors. A galvanized tubular steel frame with six chrome-finished tubular legs supports a black polypropylene bed. Steel springs are zinc finished; an elasticized frame pad is foam-padded and covered in sturdy, long-lasting black Naugahyde.

McNeil Jog-N-Tramp-38

McNeil's JNT-38 is an advanced design that promotes consistent bounce with equal spring stretch that works the jumper toward the center of the jumping area. The 16-gauge steel frame features thirty-two galvanized springs and compressed nylon spring tabs for long-lasting resilience. Resilience at the center gives the user a stronger workout—it is also safer, for obvious reasons. The heavy-duty jogging surface is weather-proof, while the spring connectors are completely concealed by a foam-padded vinyl rim cover for added safety. The entire platform rests on 6-inch polished aluminum legs with utilitarian, nonskid rubber feet.

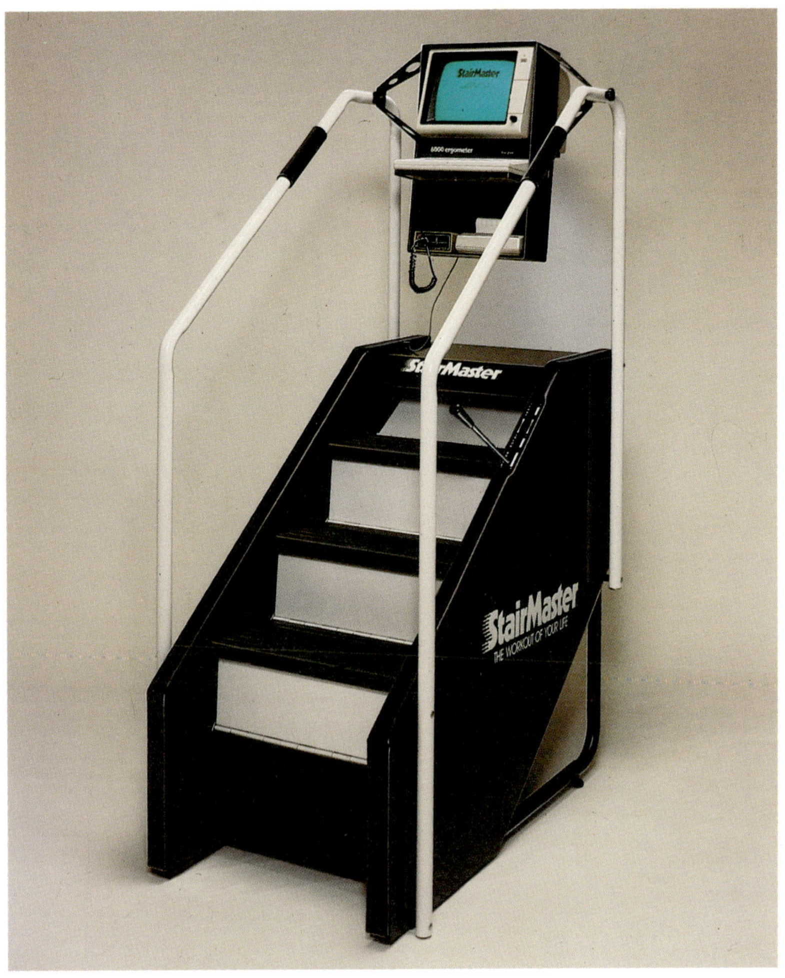

StairMaster Aerobic 5000

The StairMaster 5000 is decidedly contemporary looking with white-baked enamel handrails, metallic gray side panels, and black stair and edge guards. It features six variable climb speeds ranging from a determined walk to a brisk trot—providing an optimum workout for all ages and fitness levels. A microprocessor-controlled readout console mounted at eye level between the handrails displays such information as calories consumed, pulse rate, and flights climbed. The Aerobic 5000 shows statistics on the world's most famous vertical structures, providing the incentive for progressive exercise. Custom colors are available.

RECIRCULATING STAIRS

Stair-climbing has recently been embraced as a beneficial full-body exercise with cardiovascular as well as muscular benefits. Electronically controlled recirculating steps that descend as you climb have solved the problem of finding stairs of sufficient height to provide an uninterrupted climb. Creating an isokinetic workout, use of such machines results in monitored progressive cardiovascular and respiratory conditioning as well as muscular development of the legs, thighs, stomach, and buttocks. It is also said to improve lap times and agility for competitive athletes—all without potential damage to joints and ligaments.

When selecting recirculating stairs for the home, you should look for heavy-gauge steel construction, and lateral support wide enough to prevent wobbling. Such machines are best used as part of a more thorough conditioning program.

FREE WEIGHTS

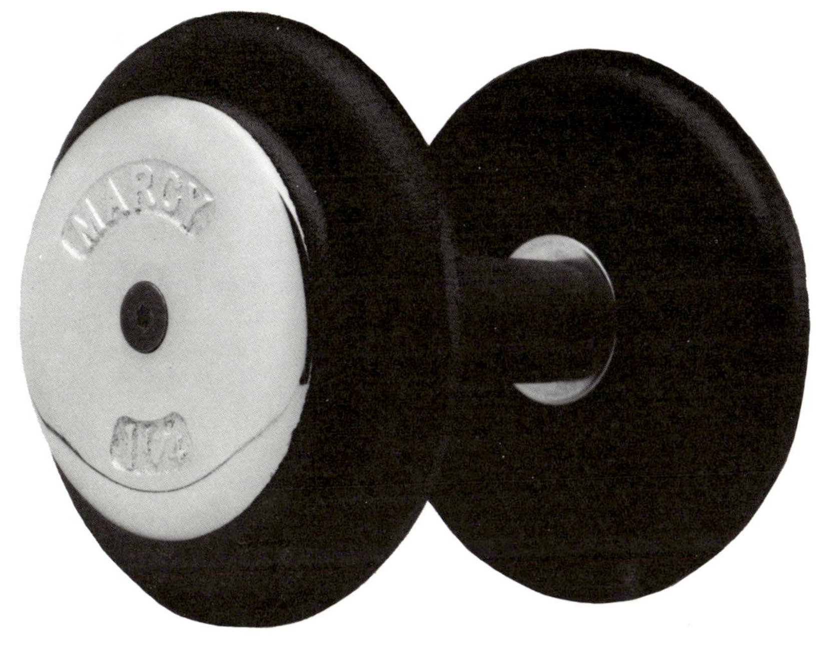

Another kind of isometric exercise is one where the muscles are exercised by resistance to weight. Weight-resistance exercise works specific muscles, but the benefit to the cardiovascular system is minimal. Weightlifting is an excellent example of this type of exercise and is ideal for improving muscular strength and local muscular endurance. Properly executed, it will also tone the muscles, provide muscle definition, and give you a more efficient body because of a greater balance between the energy required for an outcome and the outcome itself. Weightlifting can be included as an important part of the physical fitness regimen.

Generally speaking, all free weights involve various types of bars or handles that support units of weight. The selection of free weights is generally an aesthetic rather than functional choice. The weights can be cast iron or plastic; gray, chrome, black, or even gold. Cast-iron weights however, are preferable to plastic ones, which have to be larger to accommodate the same weight, take more room on the bar, and are not so accurate.

Individual weights (or plates) are generally held in place and fastened to the bar by removable collars. A variety of different bars is available, each one specifically designed to pinpoint the training of particular muscles. They are the dumbell handle, long barbell, the tricep bar, and curl bar.

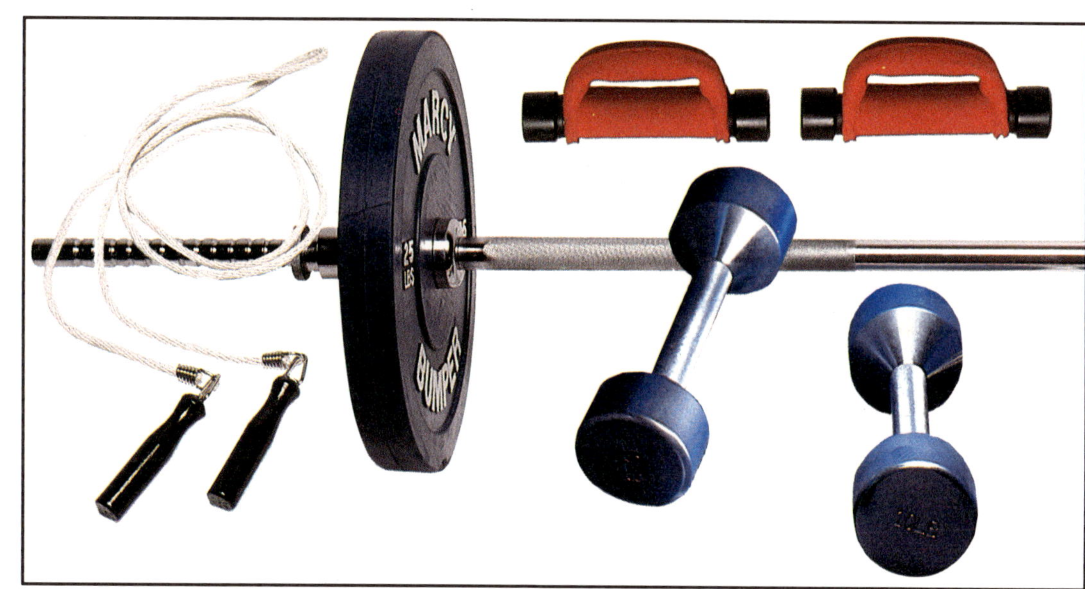

Barbells

A standard lifting bar is generally a 5 x 1-inch length of solid steel tubing used to support a fixed or variable weightload. It is the basic piece of equipment for the great variety of exercises available in free weight programs. The bar may or may not have a revolving sleeve between the individual weights and the collars to secure the plates can be welded or removable. A series of ridges (knurls) on the bar's surface allow a more positive grip.

Dumbbells

These are essentially scaled-down barbells, and consist of a small steel bar with extruded weightloads at each end. A full dumbbell program develops the upper body (triceps, biceps, shoulders, and pectorals) and generally calls for the dumbbells to be worked simultaneously, as a pair. It is also recommended that any supine exercise be performed with the aid of a bench in order to allow free shoulder movements.

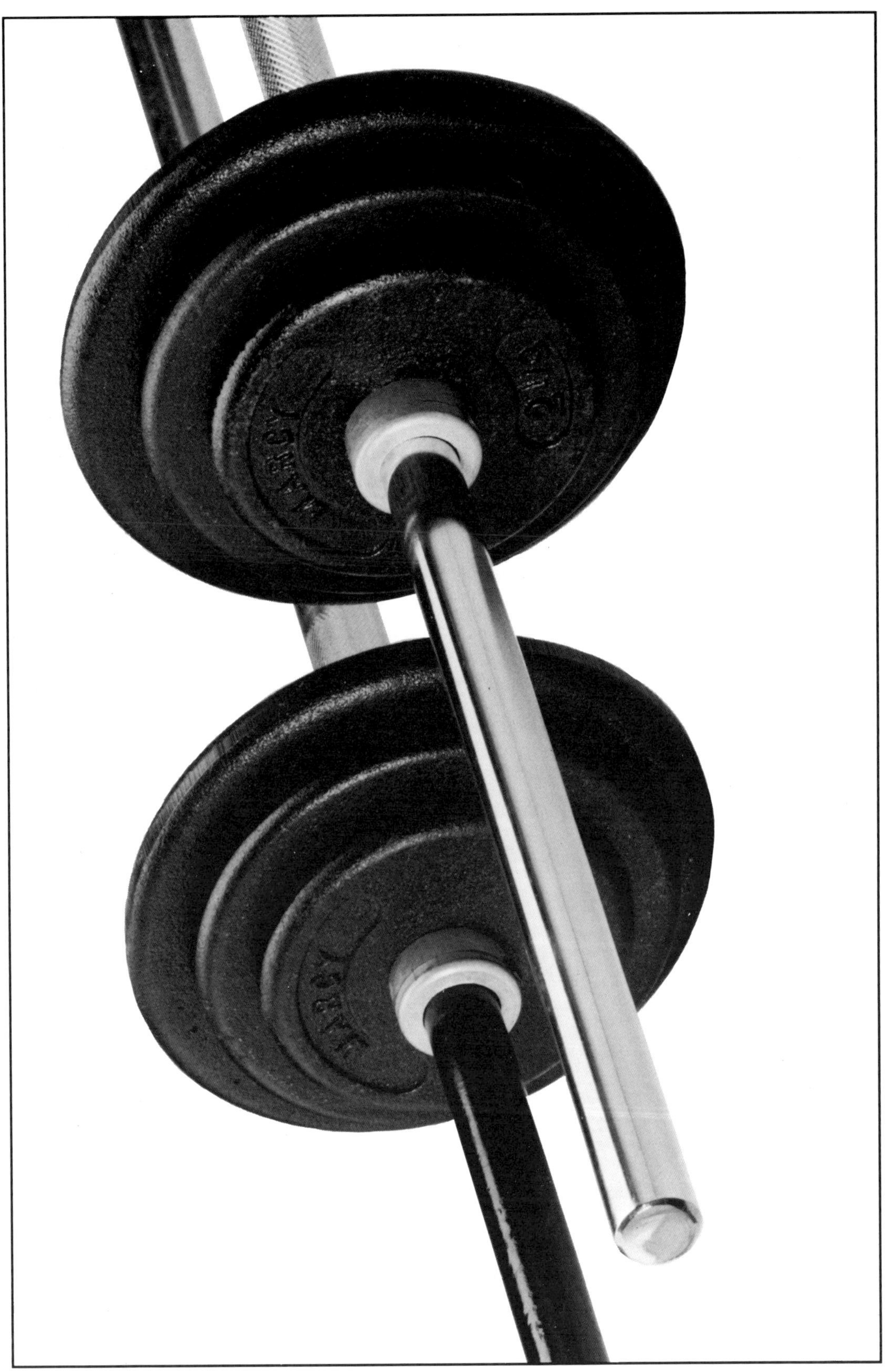

Wrist and Ankle Weights

The use of wrist and/or ankle weights can effectively distribute the workload to every part of the body. Expanding a workout among more muscles in this way will almost make the exercises feel easier, as well. Worn during work or everyday activities, the added weightload will promote muscle tone; combining them with a more concerted aerobic activity will enhance cardiovascular fitness and muscular development.

Exercise Benches

Also called supine benches, some free-weight exercise routines require special benches to provide the specific positioning needed to target certain muscles or muscle groups. The standard benches are generally 14 inches off the ground, 48 inches in length, and 18 inches wide. They generally feature a vinyl-covered, padded plywood top on a heavy-gauge steel support frame and legs. A supine bench press rack—in combination with the standard bench—provides adjustable weight cradles upon which to rest the barbell and weights and gives more options in the exercise routine, as well as a safety control factor. The better racks provide as many as four starting heights, with the uppermost prongs being the correct starting height for a seated military press.

Marcy Fixed Weight Barbell

The Marcy Type A Fixed Weight Barbell is of 82,000 PSI cold-rolled steel, with a deluxe chrome-finish, with precision knurled grips and four aluminum collars. The Type B model is of 69,000 PSI hot-rolled steel finished in black lacquer, with chromed revolving center sleeve. It also features welded inner and aluminum outer collars. The barbell's weight plates are black-lacquered.

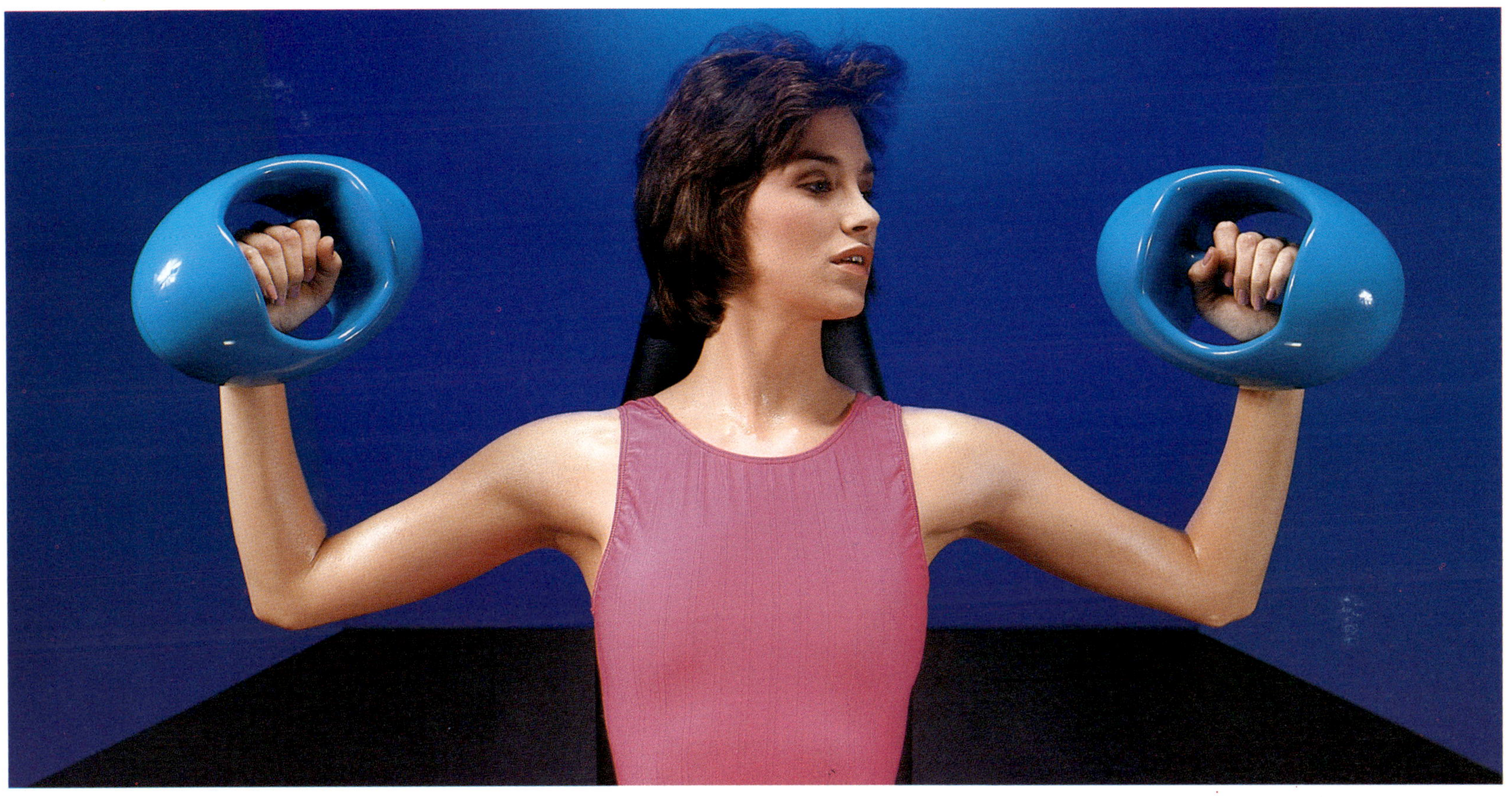

Space Weights' molded plastic-shell design offers the user free weight flexibility with a stylish new outlook. Individual weight loads are controlled by filling each hollow shell with either water, sand, or lead shot.

DP Curl Bar

The curl bar is a specially designed support bar used to work the forearm muscles. It is approximately 5 inches in length and is available in either solid or tubular steel. The center of the bar is slightly bowed, allowing for greater proximity to the body; flanking this central bend are two additional, smaller bends for placement of the hands. These allow for maximum tension on the forearms when executing a curl. To hold the weights in place, the bars come with either four collars (two inside and two outside) or with two welded inside lips and two removable collars.

DP Tricep Bar

The tricep bar is a small tubular steel lifting bar with an oval-shaped, bifurcated midsection. Two parallel steel handgrips span the open midsection, helping to establish the correct hand/arm posture for an effective shoulder/arm program. Weight plates are secured on the bar by removable collars.

Huffy 110lb Barbell Set Model 7400

Generally free weights can be purchased as a set that can include bars, sleeves, collars, and weights. The Huffy 110lb Barbell Set Model 7400 comes with a 5-inch steel lifting bar and deep-knurled chrome-plated revolving sleeve. Four collars are also supplied: two inside collars with set screws and two outside collars with quick-release handle bolt wrench. There are also two dumbbells complete with two chrome-plated revolving sleeves and four dumbbell collars. The weights are cast iron and are provided in the following increments: two 6-kilo (13-pound) plates; four 4-kilo (9-pound) plates; four 2-kilo (4½-pound) plates, and four 1-kilo (2-pound) plates. A training chart also comes with the set. Other manufacturers also offer such complete sets; all manufacturers, including Huffy, offer less expanded versions.

Space Weights

Space Weights by Grafar Corp. feature a unique design concept which enables the user to progress from a 1¼-pound (1-kilo) to a 25-pound (11-kilo) weightload, all while using a single molded plastic shell. Fabricated in high-impact plastic, football-shaped, hollow shells can vary in weight, depending on the material used to fill them. Unfilled, the shell weighs 1¼ pounds (½ kilo), a good starting weight for some exercise therapies and a convenient travel weight. Filled with water, the unit weighs 5 pounds (2 kilos); with sand, 7½ pounds (3½ kilos); and with lead shot, up to 25 pounds (11 kilos). More versatile than conventional dumbbells, Space Weights's unique design enables them to be easily slipped on your ankle for an infinite number of leg exercises as well. Space Weights are currently available in high-gloss red, blue, or yellow finish.

This Marcy incline bench features a chrome finished leg curl attachment with padded ankle rollers. The user can vary the resistance by sliding additional weight plates onto a pair of extruded steel pins located on either side of the leg curl's axle. Leg curl routines are commonly performed in a prone position, either on one's stomach or back.

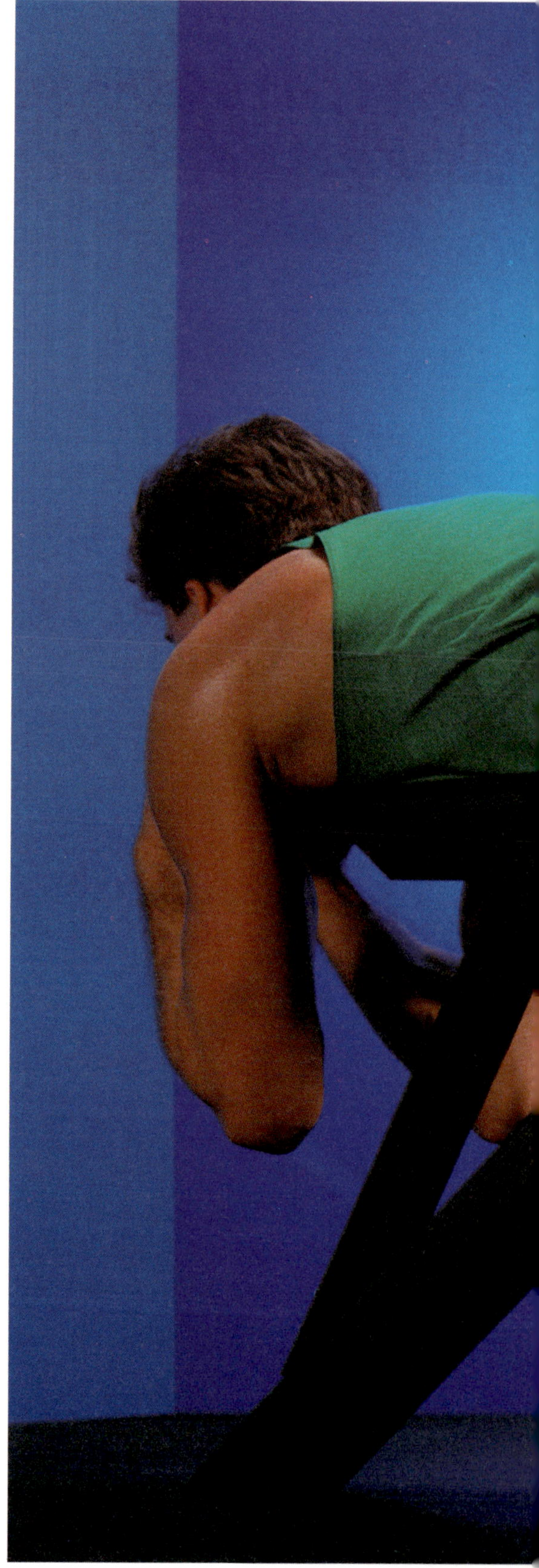

Marcy Deluxe Low Bench 1245

Marcy's Deluxe Low Bench features a satin-finish chrome frame, unique dual-support T-leg design, and a black cushioned seat. The 30-ounce backed vinyl upholstery and 2-inch-thick padding are affixed to a 1-inch-thick plywood base, the underside of which is varnished. Heavy-gauge 2½-inch-thick steel box tubing is used for the frame and legs. The term "low" is merely a generic term used by most manufacturers.

Huffy Pulley Bench Model 575

The Huffy Pulley Bench is distinctively styled with a high-gloss black tubular steel and chrome frame. The bench is covered in padded black vinyl and features a unique incline adjustment mechanism. The chrome-finish leg curl features padded ankle rollers and, conveniently, will accept any weight plate, including those of other manufacturers, with a 1-inch bore. The chrome weight cradles are also adjustable to a variety of starting heights. The overhead pulley support rack allows the option of additional exercise routines, using stacked weight plates and the dial hand stirrups.

Marcy Standard Low Bench 1240

The Standard Low Bench by Marcy also features a black cushioned seat, but with the more conventional round steel tubing for frame and legs. Tested for up to 1,000 pounds, the standard model comes with a ½-inch-thick plywood top and backed vinyl upholstery. Legs are designed with a wide stance for extra lateral stability. This is essentially a deluxe version of the 1245 model, with heavier-gauge materials which should last longer and withstand, presumably, greater wear and tear.

Marcy Incline Bench 1920

An incline bench is ideal for specialized conditioning of the pectoral, deltoid, and bicep muscle groups. The 1920 by Marcy is a sleek design: tapered black cushion and satin chrome frame. A plywood board with radius corners upholds 30-ounce, backed and padded vinyl upholstery. Heavy duty 2½-inch tubular steel uprights support the bench and the contoured footplate is solid steel. The incline bench puts the user in a most advantageous posture for the performance of particular routines. An alternative would be to lie on the floor, which would inhibit movement.

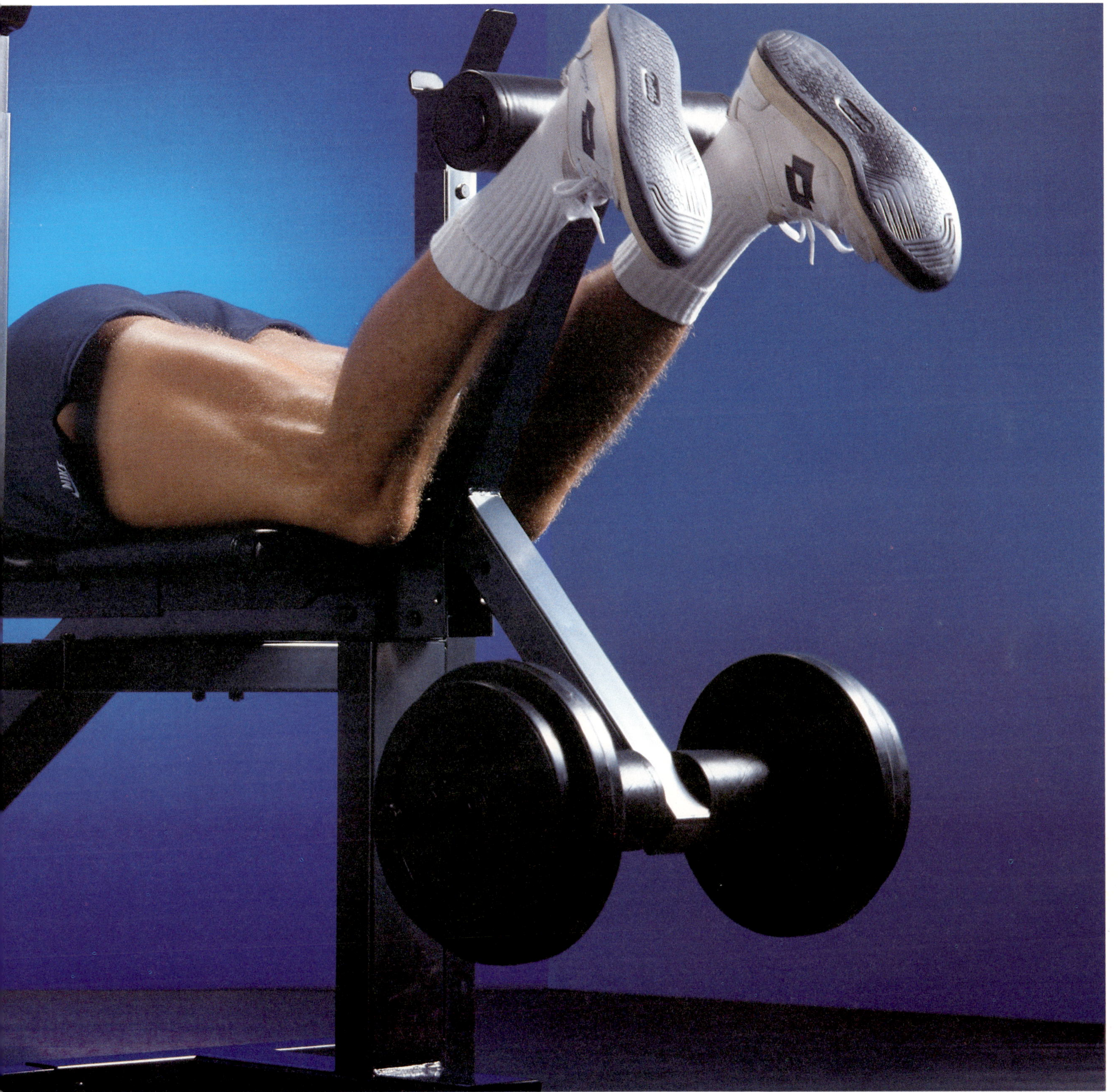

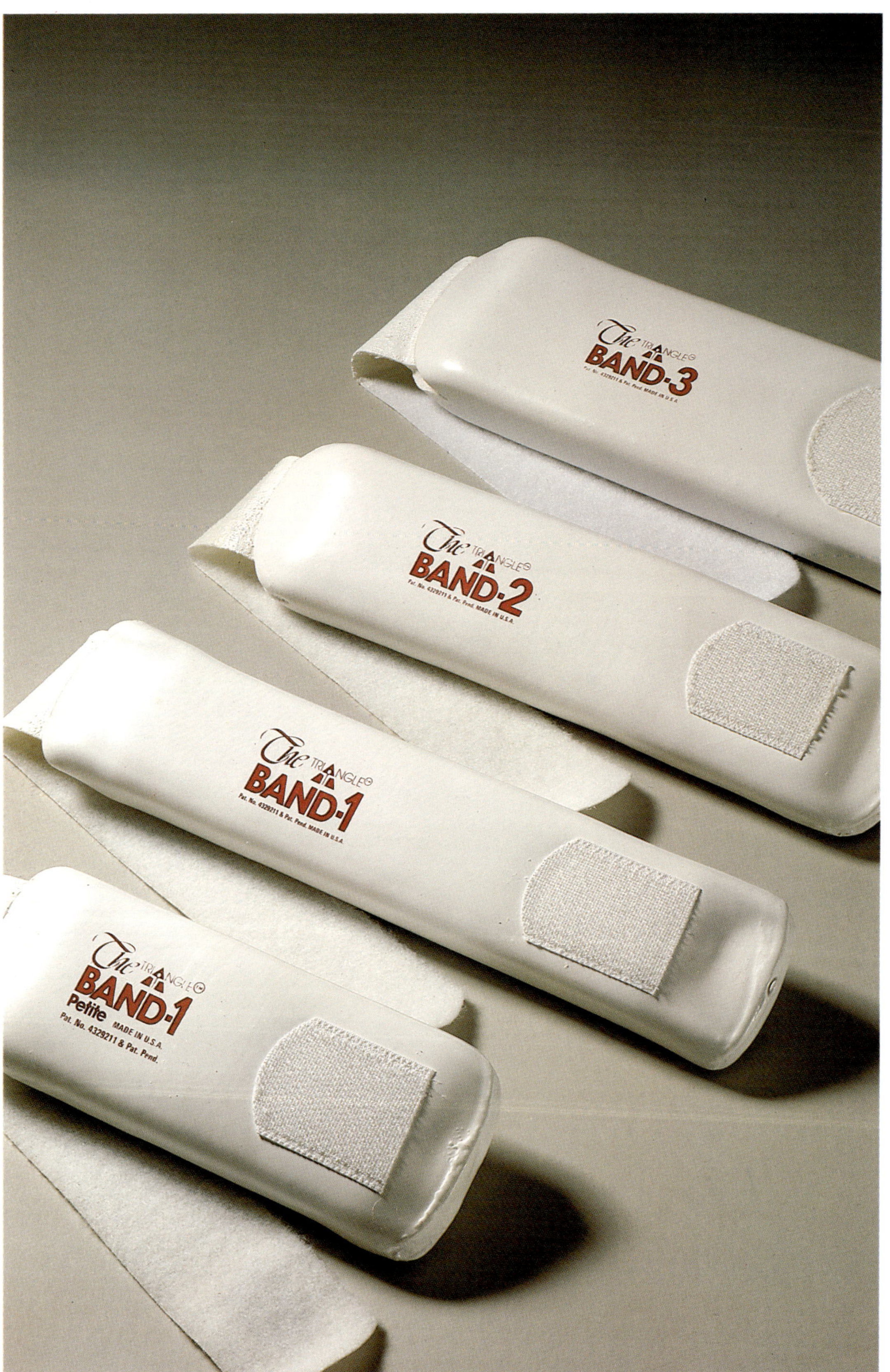

When attached to the user's extremities, wrist and ankle weights can enhance the efficiency of any stretching, bending, or aerobic exercise routine. Especially suited to leg flexion exercises, the individual weight loads can be increased as the user progresses.

Pennypak Wrist and Ankle Paks

Pennypak Products makes variable weight wrist/ankle paks with a rather unique approach—pennies are used to obtain the exact amount of weight desired. Loose pennies or rolls of pennies (one pound equals 150 pennies, or three rolls) are simply inserted into the pockets and sealed with a Velcro fastener. This is a nifty gimmick. The paks are interchangeable: They can be used on the wrist or ankle. Size is dependent on weight capacity. All colors are currently offered in four weight capacities: 1 pound (½ kilo), 3 pounds (1½ kilos), 6 pounds (3 kilos), and 12 pounds (5½ kilos).

The paks are constructed of abrasion-resistant nylon with a series of pockets for the pennies. When filled, they simply wrap around the wrist or ankle and are held in place by an exterior belt with a Velcro fastener. Colors available are burgundy, royal blue, and forest green; the 1-pound model is available in silver-gray or cobalt - blue.

Triangle Band

Triangle Bands are interchangeable weighted cuffs insulated by a thick layer of soft vinyl-covered foam. Solid lead weights are linked together like a metal watchband and completely encapsulated in the foam lining. This special interlocking design ensures a perfect fit, conforming to the contour of the extremity. The weights are covered in washable white vinyl and feature an adjustable Velcro closure. They are available in three weight capacities: 1 kilo (2 pounds), 1.5 kilos (3½ pounds), and 2.0 kilos (4½ pounds). A scaled-down "petite" version, more suited to the smaller individual, is also available in 1 kilo (2 pounds).

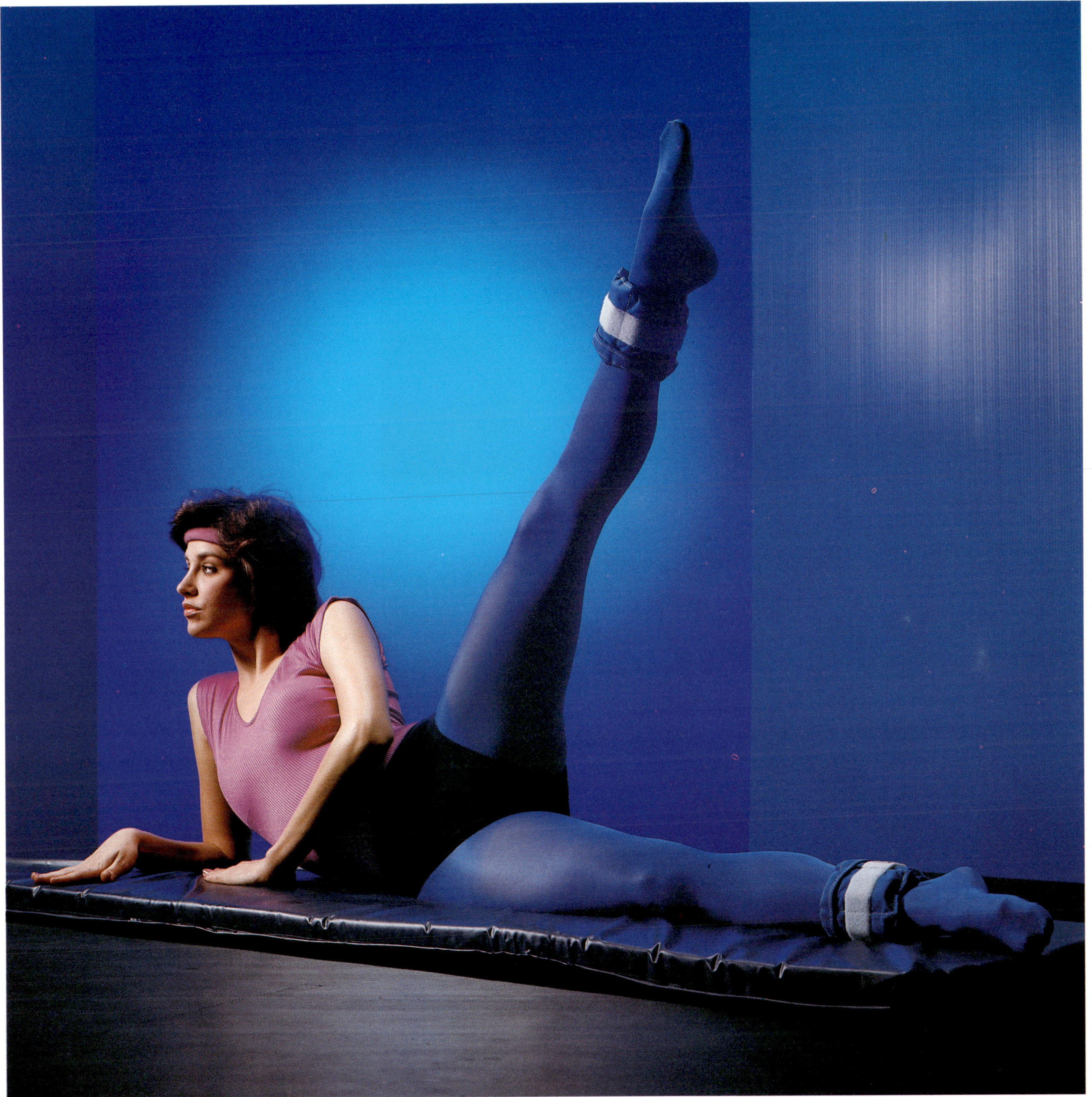

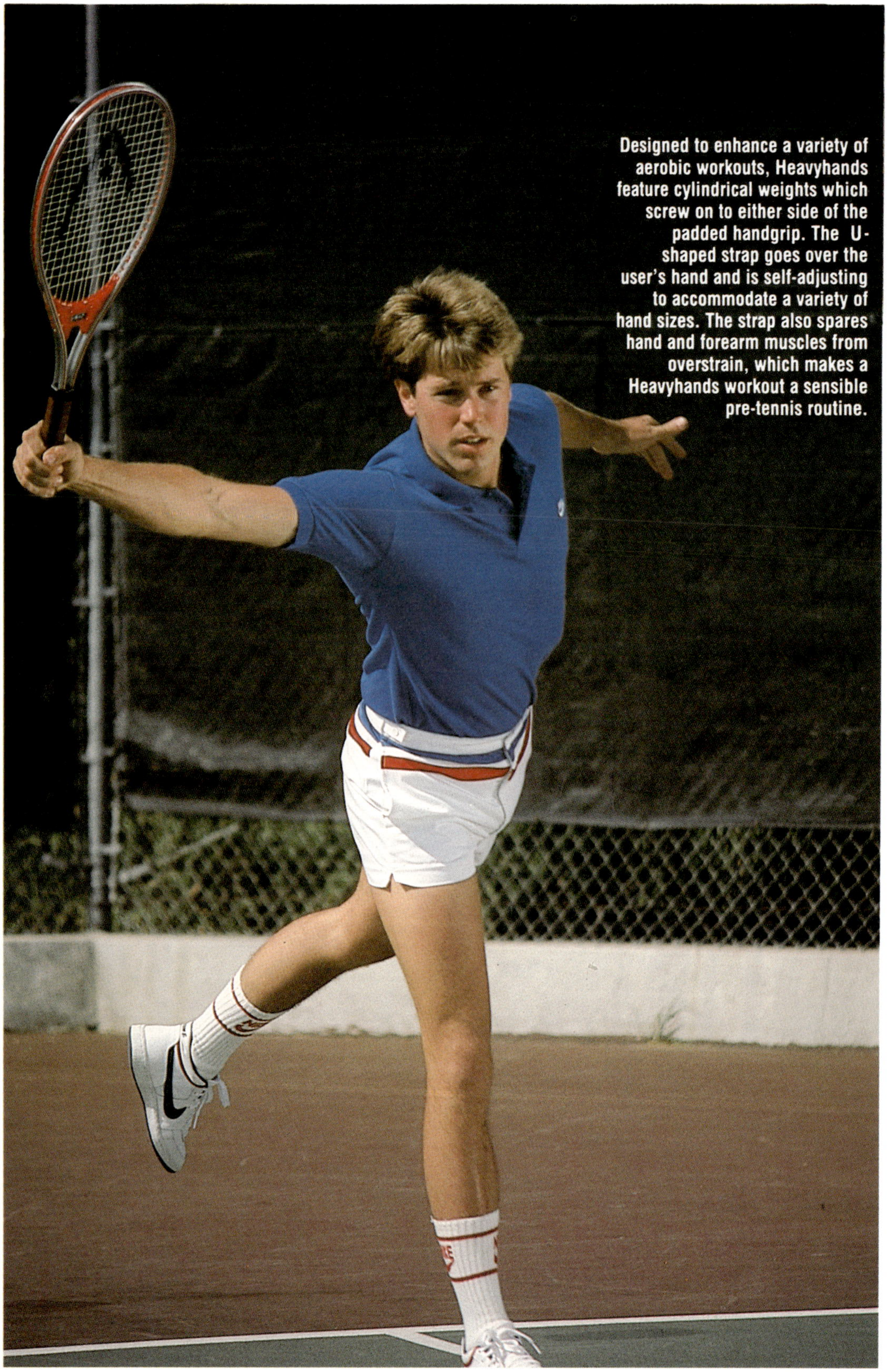

Designed to enhance a variety of aerobic workouts, Heavyhands feature cylindrical weights which screw on to either side of the padded handgrip. The U-shaped strap goes over the user's hand and is self-adjusting to accommodate a variety of hand sizes. The strap also spares hand and forearm muscles from overstrain, which makes a Heavyhands workout a sensible pre-tennis routine.

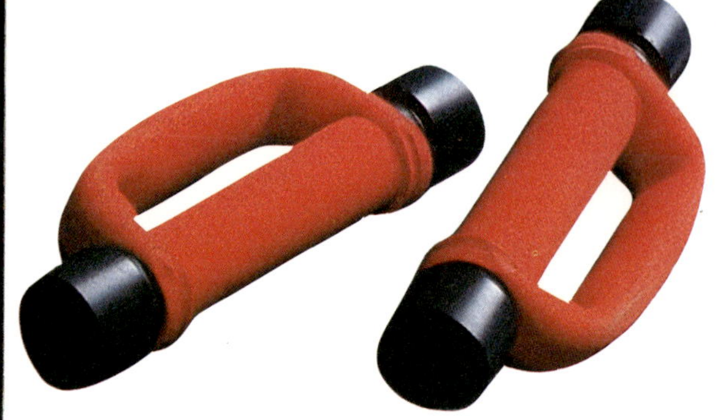

AMF Heavyhands

Heavyhands were designed with the idea of making your workout aerobically more efficient. Their unique open handle design was created to shift the stress away from the small muscles of the hand and forearm toward the more massive muscles of the upper torso.

The two-part handle design features a cylindrical handgrip, foam-cushioned for comfort, with built-in tolerances for perspiration and daily usage. The U-shaped strap, which goes over the top of the hand just behind the knuckles, is self-adjusting to accommodate hands of varying sizes and shapes. The strap also spares hand and forearm muscles from overstrain and cramping. Each grip features twin matte black cylindrical weights that screw on to either side of the handle. Heavyhands are available in 1- to 10-pound (½- to 4½-kilo) weightloads.

Handiweights

Handiweights from Ole's Innovative Sports feature innovative design and construction. Anatomically designed so that the weight is spread evenly from the wrist to the fingers, Handiweights are made of soft, malleable lead covered with soft, comfortable neoprene. A cushioned cylindrical handgrip permits a comfortably clenched fist while the rest of the "glove" covers the top of the hand, wraps around the wrist where it is fastened by a Velcro strap. All these details ensure a virtually perfect fit. The Handiweights are currently available in 2-pound (1-kilo) 4-pound (2-kilo), and 6-pound (3-kilo) versions (weight capacity per "glove," not the combined weight). Half-pound additions (up to a 2-pound maximum) can increase the workload gradually, without requiring any change to a new or heavier pair.

WEIGHTLIFTING MACHINES

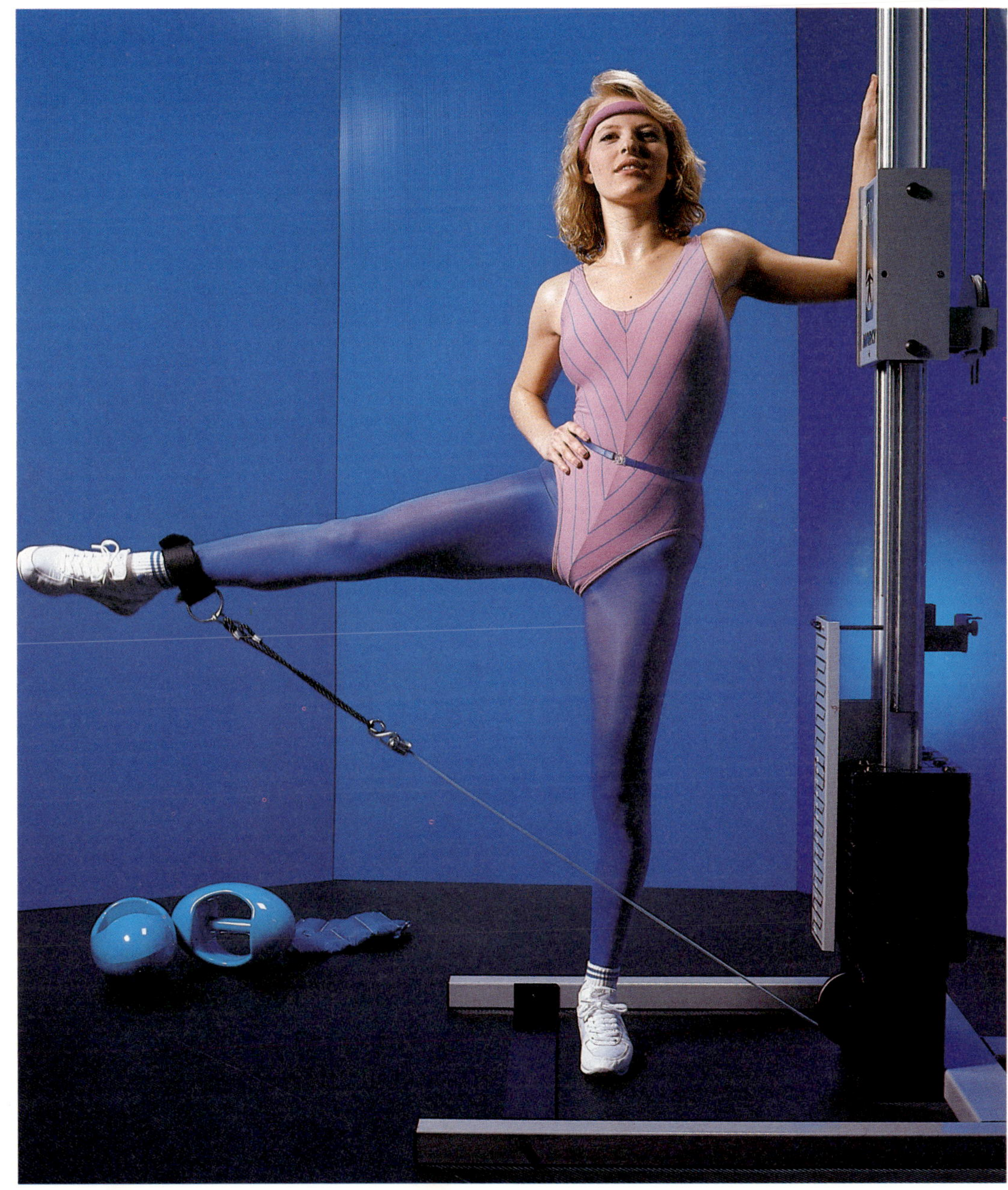

Weightlifting machines offer a safer and more convenient—albeit more expensive—alternative to lifting free weights. Most machines feature one of two techniques to provide resistance against which you push or pull: either a cable and pulley system and horizontal press bar, both attached to a captive stack of weight; or your own body weight.

A major convenience of the machines is that they are made up of one or more stations, or positions, from which different muscle groups can be worked. Depending on the exercise performed and the condition of the user, the weightload can be adjusted by simply slipping pins in and out of the weight stack. Deluxe models are equipped with multiple stations, each with its own weight stack, enabling more than one person to exercise simultaneously. Separate weight stacks also eliminate the task of "cable switching," thereby allowing for an uninterrupted and efficient work flow.

Most of these fitness machines are freestanding, although there are a number of wall-mounted versions (single weight stack) currently available. Choice of machine is limited by the amount of space available. The machines are generally available with options that extend the versatility of the machine as well as your workout. When selecting a machine for home use, look for a structurally solid support frame; cables should be nylon coated with steel rather than plastic pulleys. Weight stacks should be safely held within the frame or behind steel bars and all moving parts should, of course, operate smoothly.

The seated military bench press is just one of numerous exercise routines available to an em 1-user. The 200-pound weightload from cast-iron plates offers varied resistance in 10-pound increments. Weight options can increase the em 1's capacity to 320 pounds.

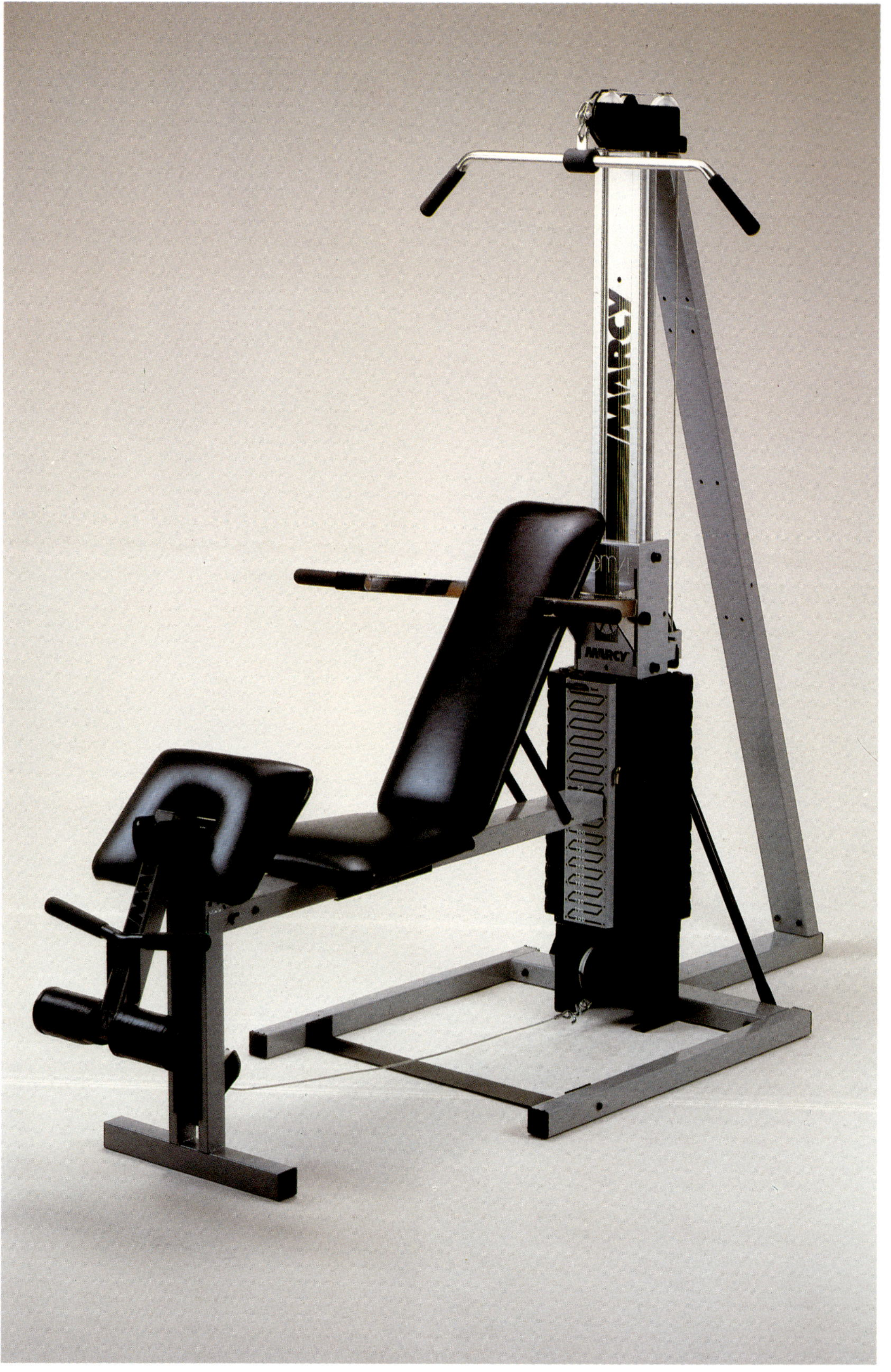

Marcy em 1

The Marcy em 1 is probably the most advanced option-assisted multiple-station home gym. It features a stylish, yet professional look with an extruded aluminum and welded steel frame finished with a gray baked-powder coat. All contact surfaces are covered in high-density foam and black backed vinyl and feature radius-cut corners. The em 1 can be wall-mounted but is also available with a free-standing accessory that allows for the attachment of a Butterfly option.

The em 1 offers 200 pounds (90 kilos) of resistance (320-pound capacity with weight options) from cast-iron plates and allows for selectorized resistance in 10-pound (4½-kilo) increments. This model comes equipped with lat bar, leg flexion/extension, arm curl, high and low pulley, single and double pulley handles, press/incline bench/abdominal board, ankle strap, and exercise chart. A leg press/squat bar is also available. Gross weight is 295 pounds (133 kilos); with freestanding option, 360 pounds (163 kilos).

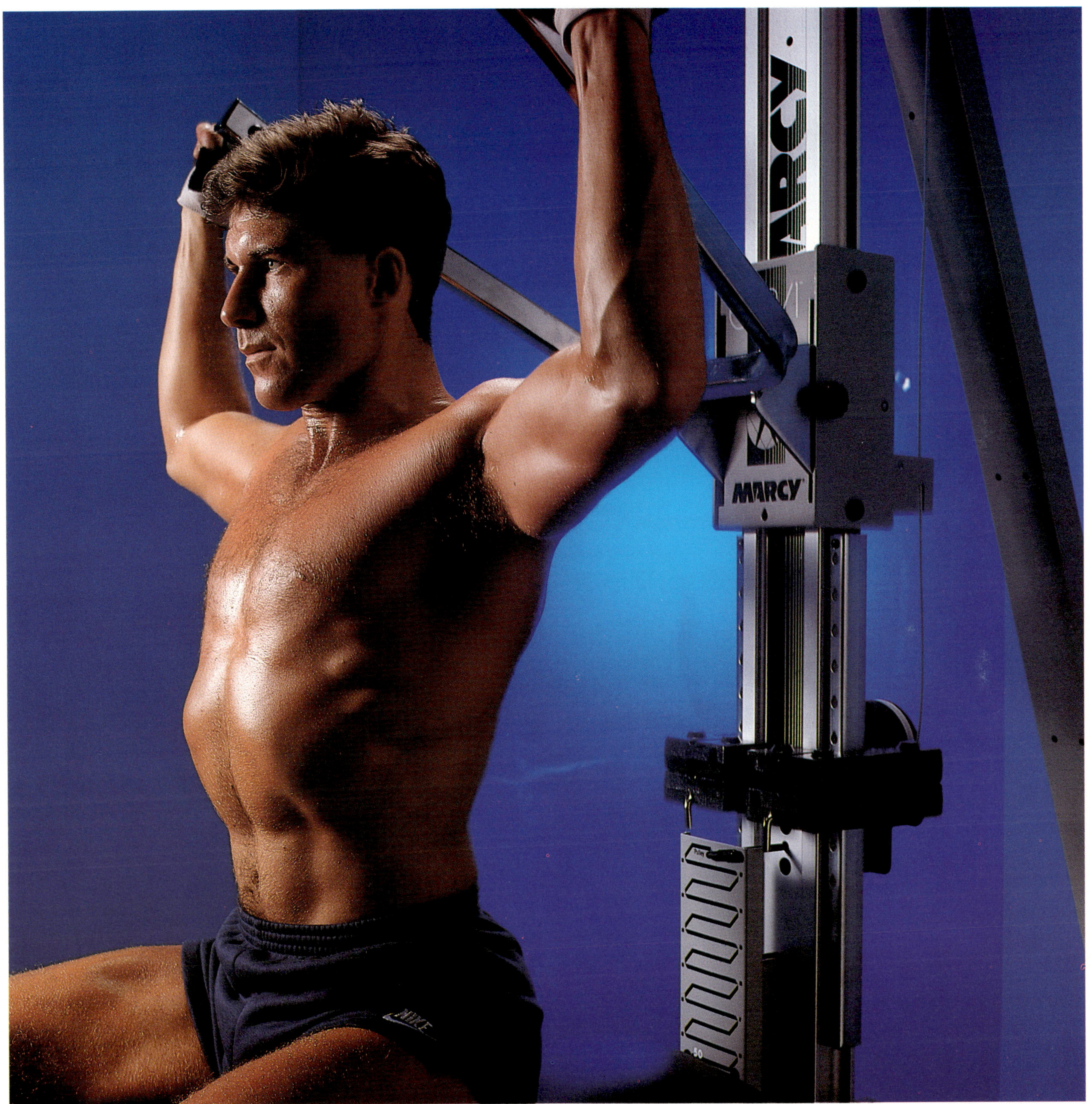
MARCY
MARCY
NIKE

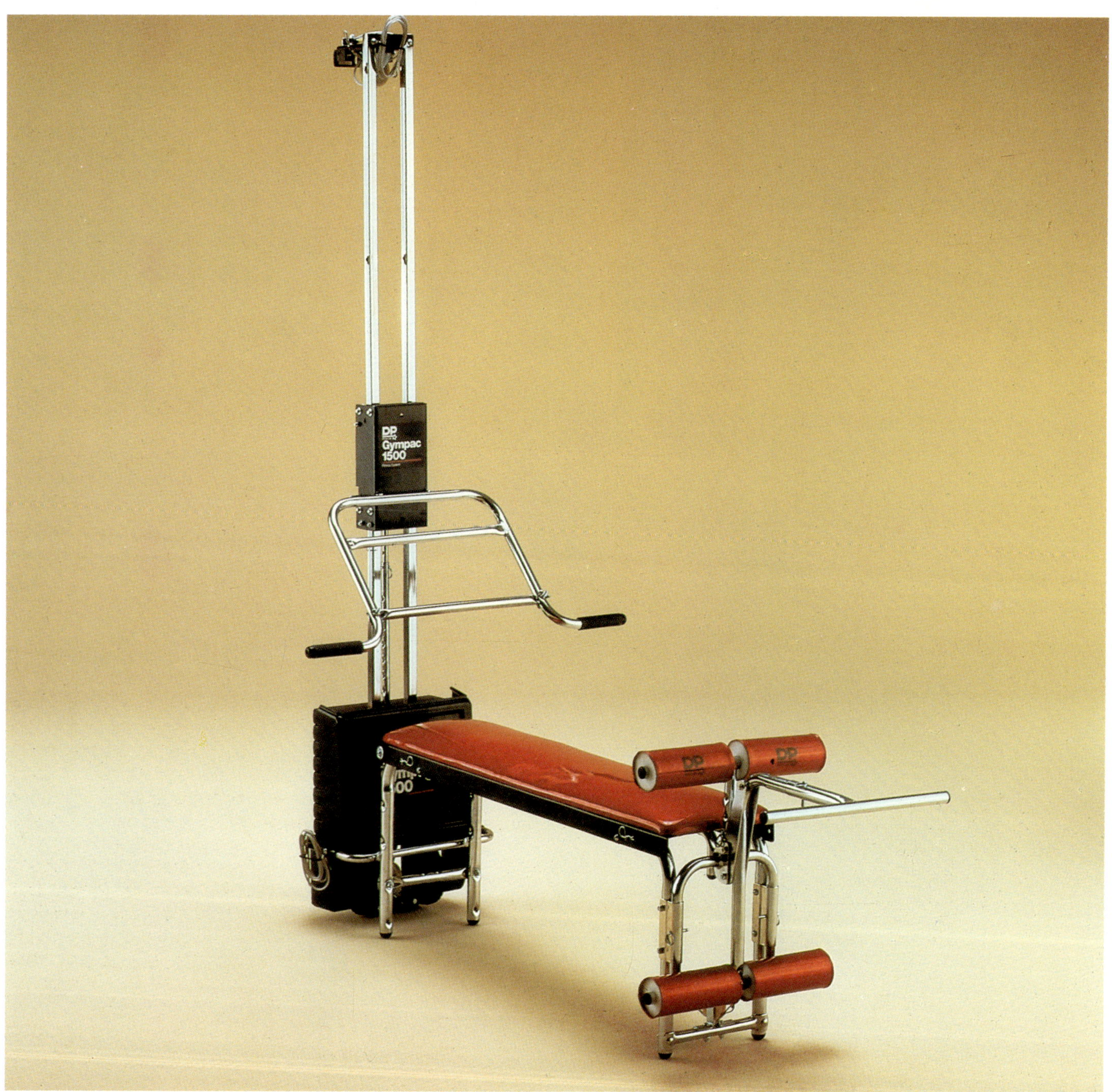

◁ **The DP Gympac 1500 is an ideal home gym suited to weightlifting, body building, athletic improvement, and general physical fitness. A matte-black weight stack and housing complement the unit's chrome-plated tubular steel frame. The DP Gympac 1500 attaches to a single wall stud and requires only three screws to mount.**

The Paramount FitnessTrainer II is a professional-looking home gym finished in heavy, bright nickel-chrome plating. The unit illustrated here shows the vertical knee raise, leg extension/leg curl, and chromed weight options. The standard FitnessTrainer features a chest/shoulder press and bench, high pulley with lat bar, low pulley with stirrups, T-bar, and ankle strap. ▷

DP Gympac 1500

The DP Gympac 1500 is a space-conscious, multistation, wall-mounted gym. Ideally suited for a complete workout, the 1500 features a single weight stack, press bar, high and low pulley, leg cuff, stirrups, and leg lift/leg curl rowing attachment. The heavy-gauge tubular steel frame is chrome-plated; the weight stack and housing are finished in matte black. Using the bench and/or the press bar you can execute a standard bench press, seated military press, double leg extension, rowing exercises, and close-gripped chin-ups. With the high or low pulley individually, a number of routines—leg raises, leg pull-down, forearm pull, and seated rowing exercise—can all be performed without difficulty.

The 1500 comes with a special wall-mounting system that includes a base plate and hanger stud bolt—all of which require only three screws. The Gympac stores completely in place against the wall occupying a height of 85 inches and a depth of 17½ inches. Easily disconnected from the wall, built-in castors expedite roll-away storage.

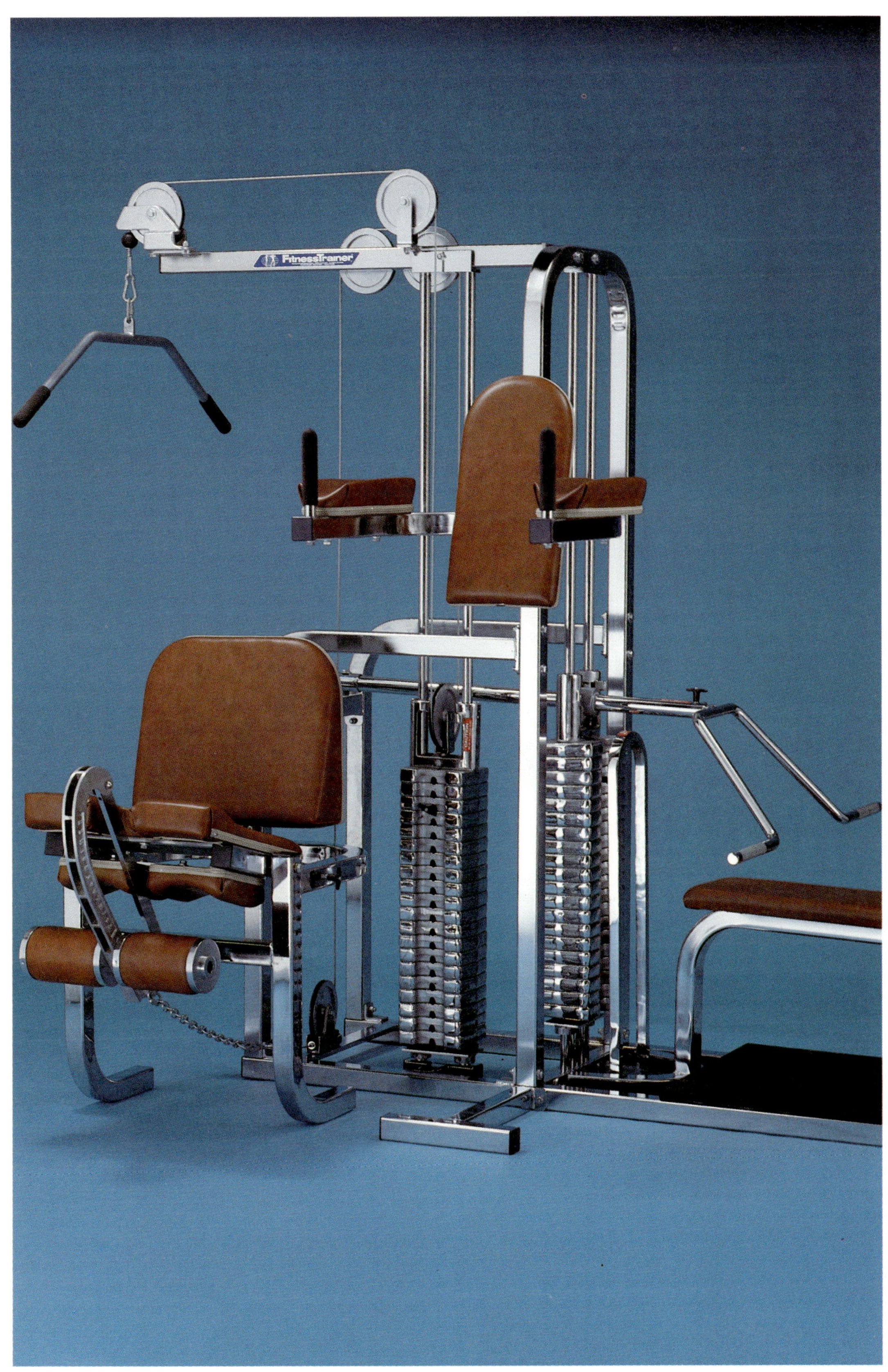

Paramount FitnessTrainer

The FitnessTrainer by Paramount is a multi-station unit with a decidedly professional appearance. The entire frame is finished in bright nickel-chrome plating, and all the contact surfaces are upholstered in heavy Naugahyde. Standard features include chest/shoulder press with bench, high pulley with lat bar, low pulley with stirrups, T-bar, and ankle strap. Options on the unit illustrated here include vertical knee raise, leg extension/leg curl, and chromed weight options. Also available are a squat option with pads, leg press, Roman bench, and sit-up board. The entire frame is heavy-gauge 2-inch steel tubing, less than 7 feet high, and is equipped with built-in safety features.

Pro Plus Exercise System

The Pro Plus Exercise System also utilizes a resistance principle. The resistance here is derived from a unique source: body weight. It is your own weight pulled up and down on the glideboard that becomes the workload. Adjusting the height of the board affects the resistance accordingly: the steeper the incline, the harder you have to work. Lowering the board reduces the resistance to a smaller percentage of your total weight.

The Pro Plus Exercise System features a sleek polished chrome-plated frame with black cushioned glideboard and accessories. The glideboard is upholstered in non-tear black vinyl and mounted on parallel steel tracks; a weight bar between the glideboard and tracks accepts additional weights. A vertical U-shaped upright supports the glideboard on any of eleven height adjustments by means of steel hooks. Attached to the top of the upright is a pulley with cable and leg cuff for inner thigh pulls. There is also a two-handed arm pulley with stirrup handles to pull you up and down on the board and for doing arm curls and butterflies. The squat stand at the foot of the board is also cushion-padded in black vinyl and used for leg presses. The entire frame is made of heavy chrome-plated steel and weights 111 pounds. Additional accessories include a curl pad, swivel foot holder, and dual-handle accessory.

SLANT (ABDOMINAL) BOARDS

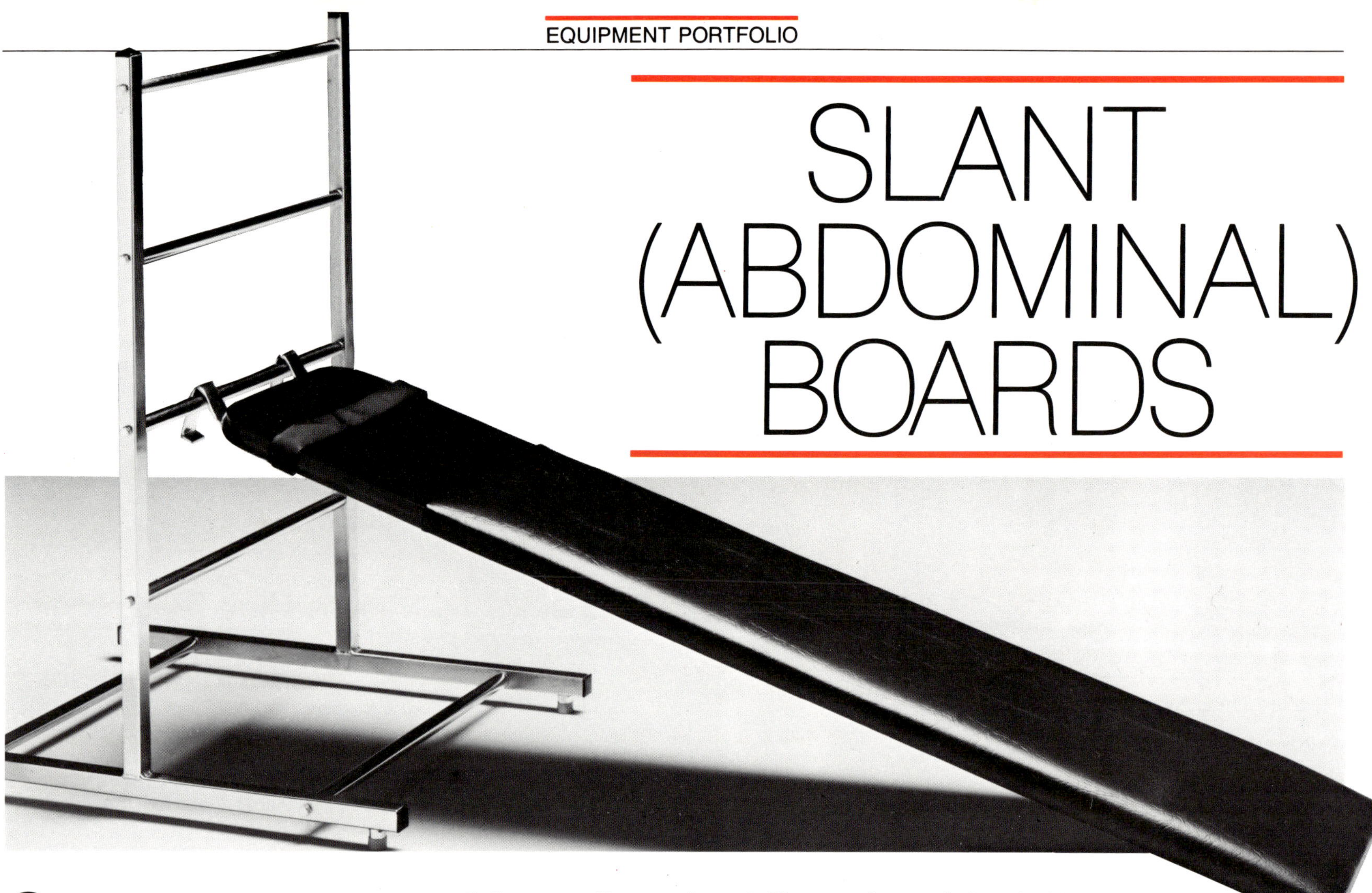

Slant boards provide improved leverage for effective abdominal conditioning. The boards are always cushioned and have a foot strap to hold you in place. Height adjustments are made by raising or lowering the board on a floor or wall ladder, which enables you to vary the performance difficulty of the sit-up or leg raise. Deluxe models are available that feature ankle rollers and handgrips to provide extra support for leg raises.

When selecting a slant board for home use, look for a solid wood base that does not buckle under weight. The board should also be thickly cushioned—to protect your back—and the upholstery should be carefully stretched and perfectly smooth. Rounded corners are an additional safety feature. Ladders should be heavy-gauge steel and should not bend under the user's weight. The vertical supports should be adequately spaced for good lateral support and should have rubber floor protectors.

Marcy Standard Board 111

The Marcy Standard Board 111 is simply styled and durable. The heart of the board is a 1½-inch thick select wood with rounded corners. The board is covered in 2-inch-thick high-density foam and heavy-gauge 30-ounce backed vinyl, shown here in black (custom colors are available). Polished steel hooks fit easily on the ladder and are widely spaced for lateral stability. A nylon web foot strap holds you securely in place and can be revolved for even wear. The board is 72 inches long, 16 inches wide, and 4 inches high.

Marcy Ladders

Marcy's floor ladders are available in four height positions. The highest is 43 inches. They are constructed of heavy-duty cold-rolled steel tubing, which is plated and buffed to a contemporary satin chrome finish. Extra-wide lateral supports ensure stability.

Tunturi Wall Board and Sit-Up Board

The Tunturi Sit-Up Board is a more pared-down version of a slant board (most of which have cushioning, for example), constructed of laminated pine. It lacks cushioning. The board features a footstrap and fastening hooks, measures 78 x 4 inches, and weighs only 20 pounds (9 kilos). A complementary wall board/minitrainer allows you to vary the height of the sit-up board as well as perform additional routines. The wall board features two vertical brackets supporting heavy-duty, horizontally arranged dowels. It measures 90 x 31 inches. Special fasteners allow for the attachment of elastic hand stirrups.

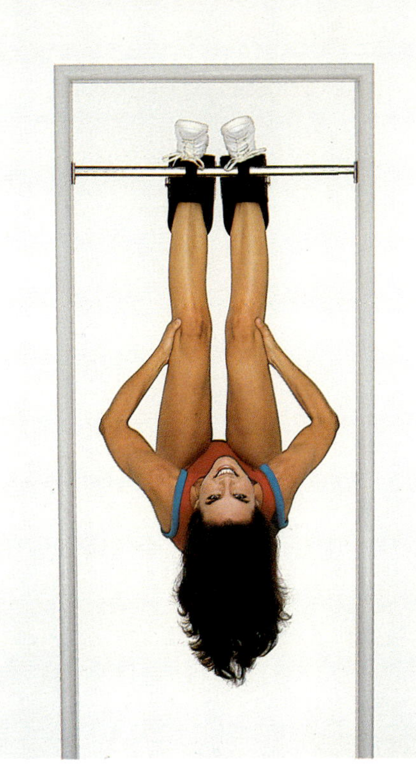

GRAVITATIONAL TRACTION

Gravity is an unrelenting force acting upon every object on earth, including the human body. Its unidirectional force guides the direction of all weight and forms stress lines to that point. When the human body is engaged in a limited occupation recreation and rest such as sitting, standing, or lying, the force of gravity can only pull the organs and tissues of the body downward. Eventually this distorts the shape of the body. Gravitational traction seeks to counter the adverse effects of gravity by a program of planned and properly guided postural exchange. Inversion machines have since been developed to meet this need. The machines essentially aid in altering and adjusting the postures of the body with respect to gravity in an effort to guide the application of gravity's molding force. The result is an alteration of the stress lines of gravity in the back, the cell walls, the organs, and the whole body, relieving and neutralizing areas of stress.

Of the six basic human postures, three produce body compression and shortening of stature (common postures), and three produce body decompression and elongation of stature (uncommon posture). The more detrimental common postures are: the erect posture, sitting and standing; the horizontal posture, lying on side, back, or front; and the flexed posture, bending forward. The uncommon postures—used to counter and correct the adverse effects of gravity produced by the common postures—are: the extended posture, bending backwards; the brachiated posture, hanging by the upper or lower limbs; and the inverted posture, standing on the hands, standing on the forearms, and hanging by the lower limbs.

When selecting a machine for home use, look for a heavy-gauge steel frame with a wide enough stance for adequate lateral support. Pivot bearings should operate smoothly and quietly and require minimum maintenance.

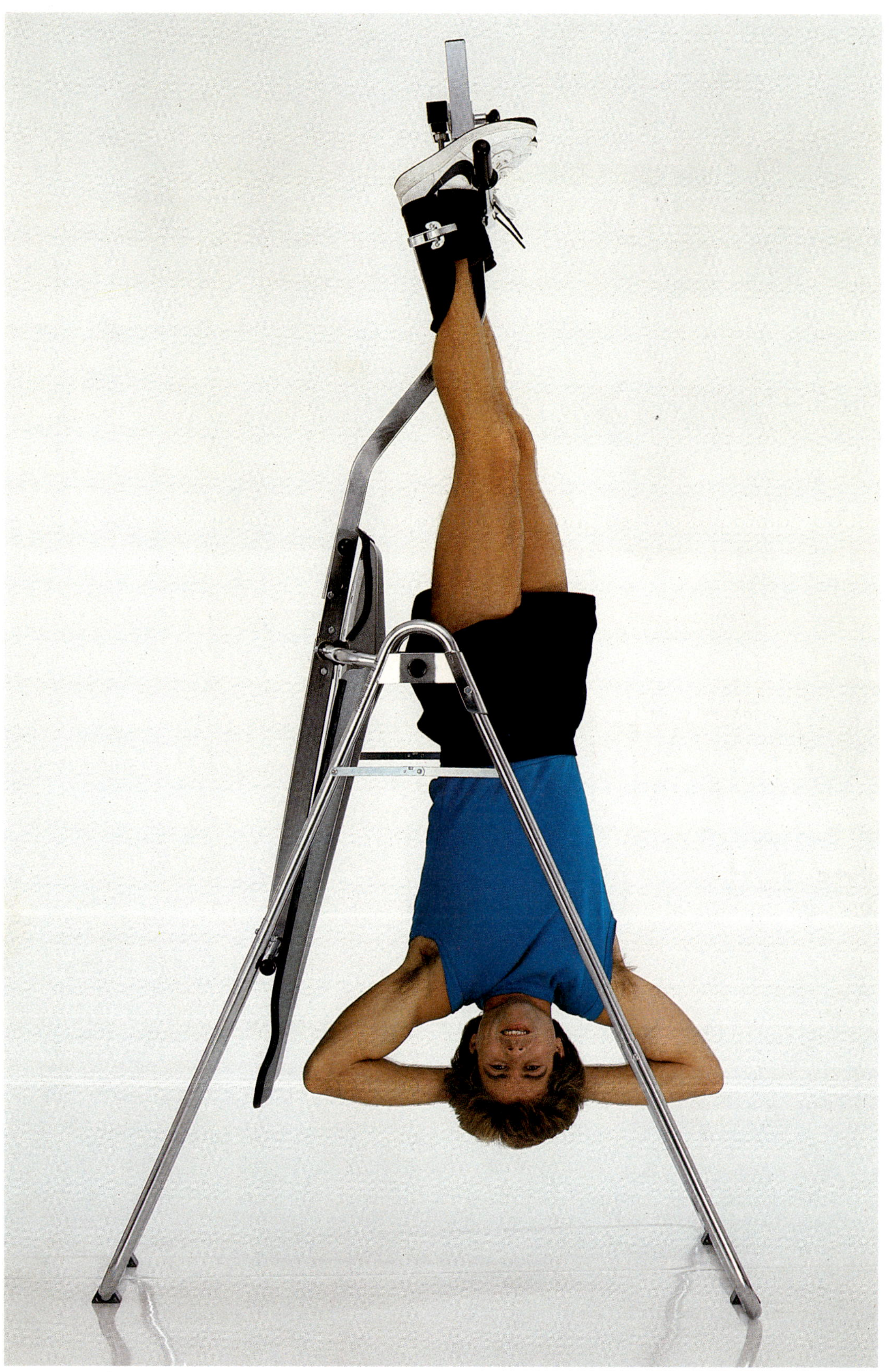

Inversion machines counter the adverse effects of gravity through a program of properly guided postural exchange. The 1150 Series offers the option of intermittent traction through oscillation (swinging) or continual traction through full inversion (free hanging) shown here. A specially patented assembly allows the user to hang freely away from the bed and locks into the inverted position.

1150 Series Gravity Guider

The 1150 Series is the most compact, economical, full-function Gravity Guider. It provides both intermittent traction through oscillation (swinging) and continuous traction through full inversion (free hanging). Well-suited for use in smaller spaces, the 1150 is foldable for easy storage and portability.

Designed with functional aesthetics in mind by Gravity Guidance, Inc., the 1-inch tubular steel frame features a matte black finish. Electrostatically applied and baked for durability, the finish is virtually chip-resistant. The contoured oscillation bed is tapered at the top and made of black nylon, which is easily removed for cleaning. The wide stance and two stabilizer bars provide maximum safety, while the specially curved footrest provides greater user control. Flushmounted hardware also improves the appearance of the machine. Convenient height and weight adjustments for individuals from 5′ to 6′6″ tall and from 100 to 300 pounds make the 1150 ultimately versatile. Gravity Boots ankle holders are available as options.

SUPPLEMENTAL EQUIPMENT

There is a wide assortment of physical fitness equipment available that does not replicate activities normally performed outdoors such as bicycling, rowing, or jogging. Grouping such equipment together, as it is here, allows for greater examination of their individual uses and benefits as well as a clearer picture of how they might fit into a program of regular home use.

Most of the equipment contained in this section is smaller, more portable, and less costly than the equipment previously discussed, and the pieces are more commonly used as part of a more comprehensive program or as an adjunct to other equipment. The combination of equipment chosen depends on such variables as sex, age, goals, current level of fitness and, of course, spatial restrictions.

Orthopod Gravity Traction System

The Orthopod is a home gravity traction system that provides an ideal position for bilateral back and abdominal exercises. It is primarily for the execution of such exercises as the forward stretch, similar to the sit-up; the backward stretch, similar to the reverse sit-up; and the torsion exercise, which is a rotary movement of the spine.

The Orthopod's unique arching/contracting action concentrates gravity resistance on the spine rather than the ankles. The machine features a pivoting pelvic/leg support mechanism set at the apex of an inverted V-shaped open frame. Fabricated in heavy-gauge tubular steel, the frame is available in either black powder coat paint or chrome-polished to a satin finish. Engineered for precision balance, the pelvic support pivots on large 2¼-inch-diameter bearings; both the pelvic and leg supports are heavily padded (a choice of colors is available) and comfortably contoured. The entire system requires only a 24 x 30-inch space and is collapsible.

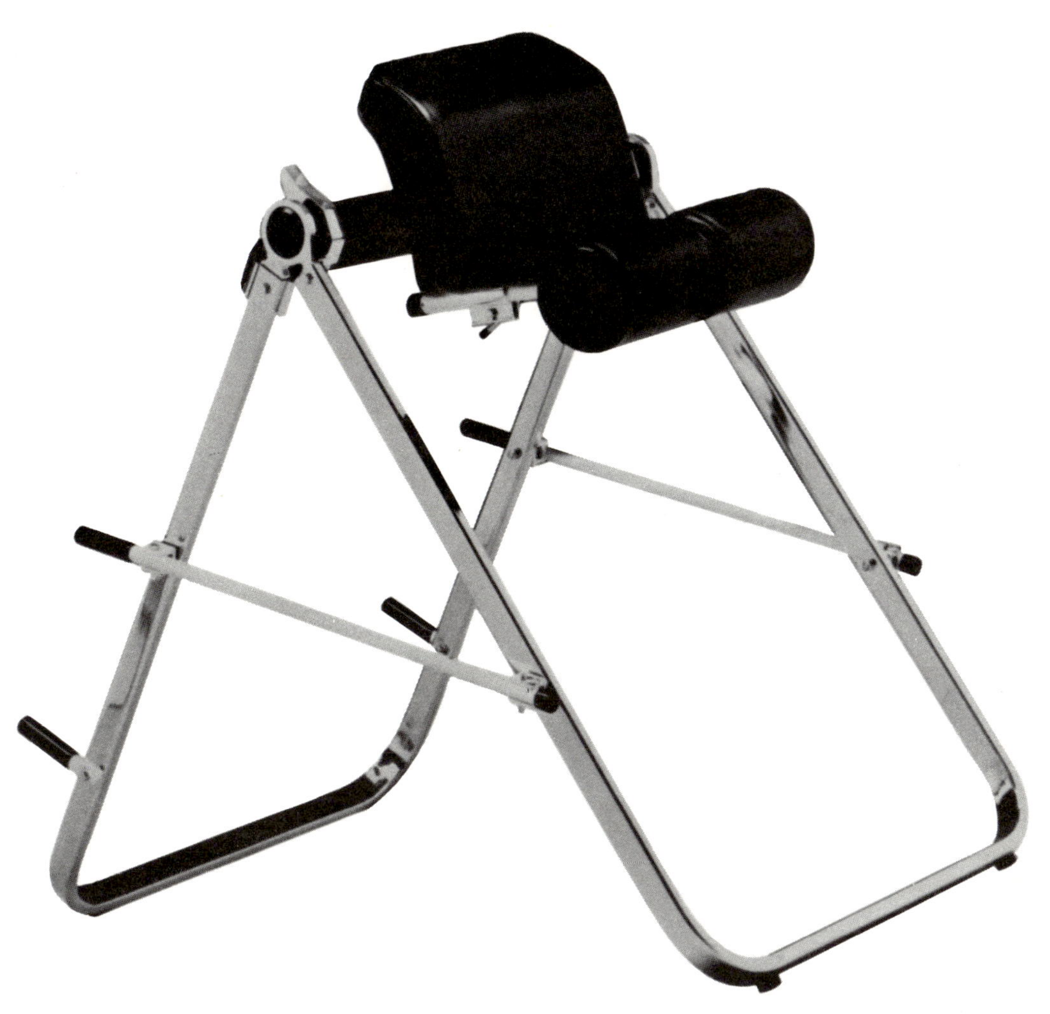

Nautilus Lower Back Machine

The Nautilus Lower Back Machine was designed solely to work the *erector spinae*—the critical muscle mass in your lower back that helps support the spine. Proper use of the machine will help strengthen the muscle, increase its flexibility, and help reverse the ill effects of bad posture, tension, and spinal compression caused by gravity.

The Nautilus Lower Back Machine offers two features that ensure beneficial results: First, the machine's resistance is always perpendicular to your spine, and since the vector of resistance moves with you, there are never any forces pressing down on you; second a unique arrangement of cams provides variable resistance to match the strength curve of a specific muscle through its entire movement.

The Nautilus Lower Back Machine features a heavy chrome-plated tubular steel frame with all contact surfaces cushioned in thick, black Naugahyde. A molded black base is stepped back (recessed) and offers the user an option of three stance heights. The entire machine measures 54 x 31 x 34½ inches and weighs 150 pounds (68 kilos). Using the machine is rather easy: Sit on the stationary inclined seat and push the movement arm by leaning back as far as possible through a 70 degree range of motion. Nine tension settings, from mild to strenuous, let you increase the load gradually as your back grows stronger. Depending on your strength, choose a milder tension to start.

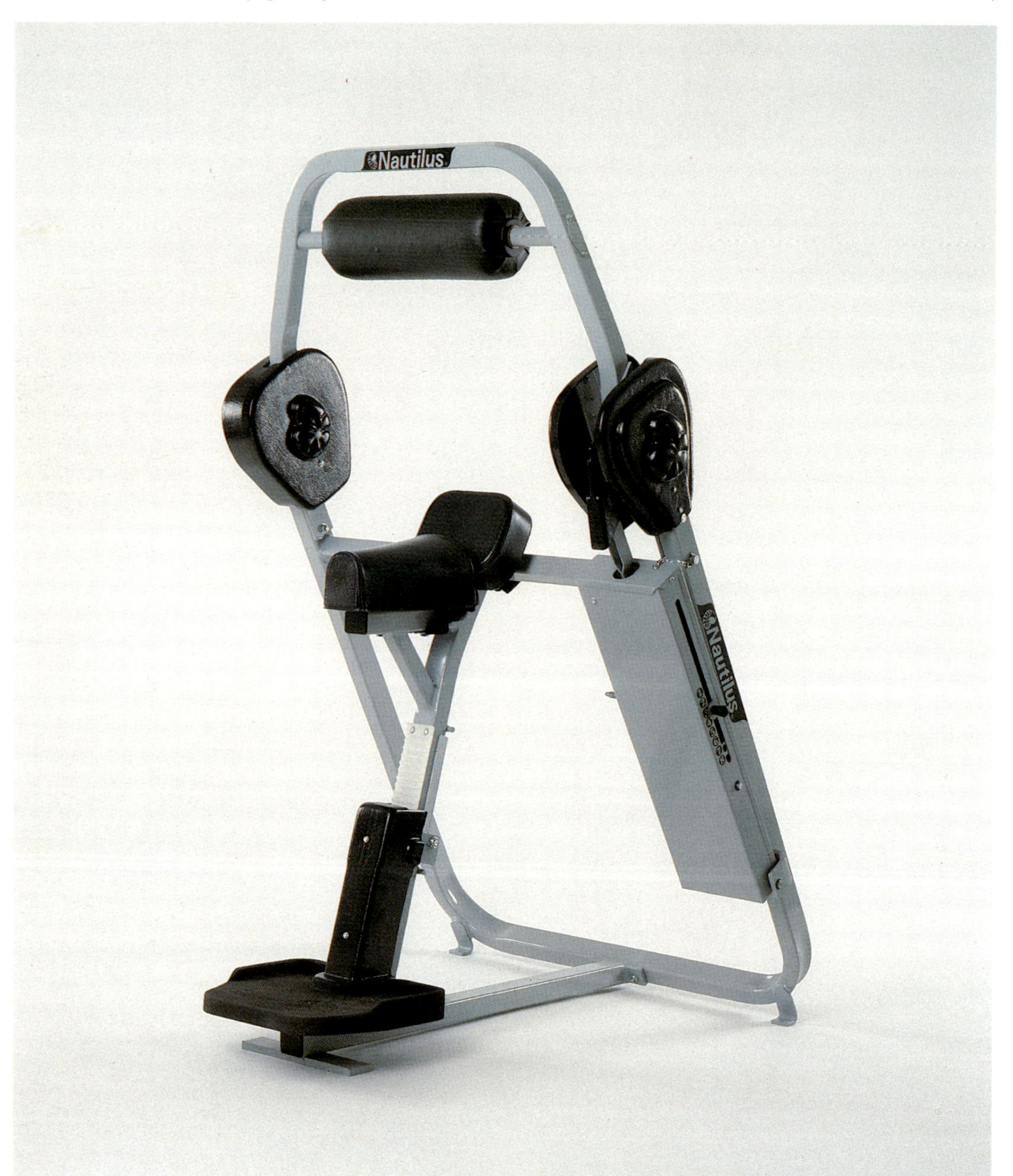

The Nautilus Lower Back Machine was designed to benefit specifically the muscles of the lower back that help support the spine. As with all Nautilus equipment, this unit is safe and easy to use: A unique system of nautilus-shaped cams provide variable resistance while the machine's vector of resistance always moves with the user.

AMF Gym Bars

The gym bar is another piece of equipment that uses your body weight as the workload (see Pro Plus Exercise System on page 35). Used as a chinning bar, it helps develop the chest, shoulders, and entire upper body while it strengthens the arms. A bar workout should include pull-ups, chin-ups, leg raises, as well as any number of gymnastic routines, depending on the bar's clearance.

AMF adjustable gym bars include exercise guides for a variety of activities from sit-ups to pull-ups. Both the DGB40 (adjusts to a 40-inch length) and the DGB (adjusts to a 32-inch length) are made of heavy-plated steel with rubber ends for tight mounting. Included in the kit are metal safety brackets.

AMF Home Exercise Mat

An exercise mat is a logical first purchase—or eventual addition—for a home gym. The AMF Home Exercise Mat is intended for such common exercises as sit-ups, push-ups, leg lifts, and tumbling. The mat is nonfolding and is available in either navy suede expanded vinyl or light blue vinyl. It measures 2 x 6 x 2 inches and is filled with a 2 -inch thickness of urethane foam.

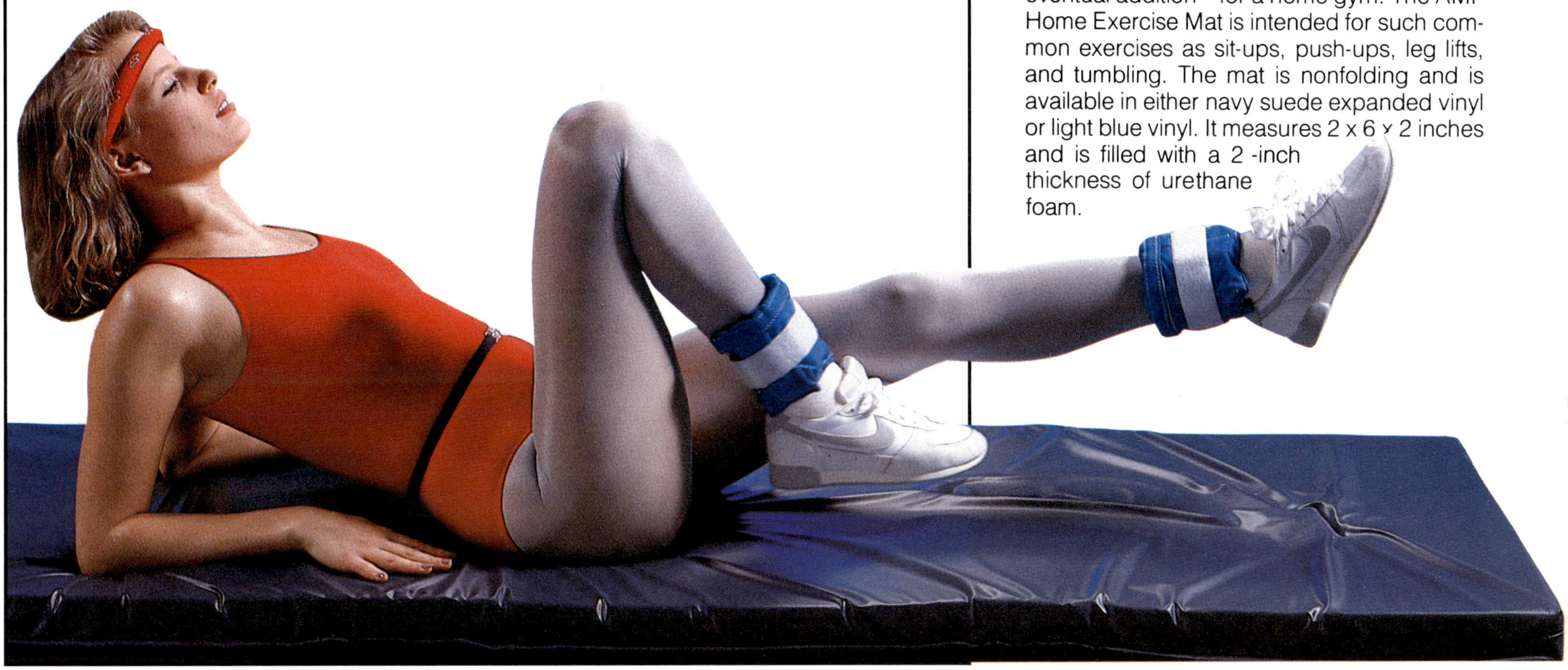

AMF Chest Pull

Chest expanders are rather elementary pieces of equipment, used for localized muscular development in the chest and shoulders. The most common chest expanders feature either cotton-wrapped cables or heavy-duty spring wire strung between two stirruplike handles. The cables or springs are removable on the better quality models.

The AMF Chest Pull comes in five models (Nos. 15, 30, 50, 31, 51) that range from three to five springs with heavy or extra-heavy tensions. All models include patented contoured handles for sure grip, and rubber shock cords. Extra springs are available for the 30ES and 31ES models.

A variety of exercises can be performed with the expander, but they are all based on the same basic movement: The user slowly stretches the expander as far as he or she is capable and either holds the outstretched position or slowly releases it. The action can be repeated in sets of ten pulls.

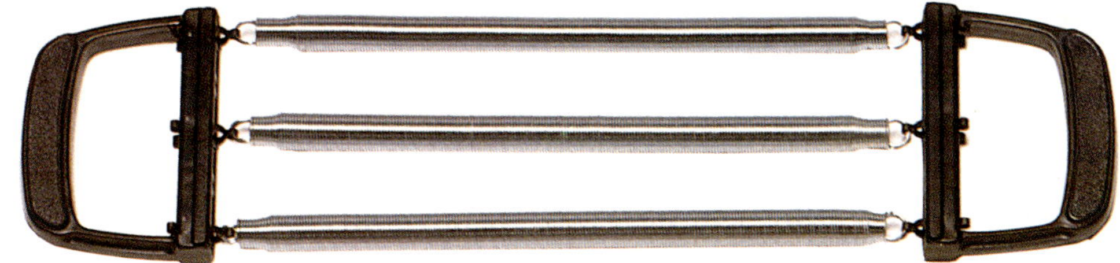

DP Extra Heavy Tension Handgrips 10-0201

Grip developers are elementary resistors used to strengthen one's grip, exercise the joints in the hand, and, to a lesser extent, work the forearm muscles. Small and lightweight, they are definitely the most covenient and portable type of fitness equipment. The user squeezes the grips together—sometimes holding them compressed for a set period—and then releases. The more common variety features a twisted, chrome-plated spring inserted between a pair of cushioned or pvc (polyvinyl chloride plastic) handles.

DP's Extra Heavy Tension Handgrips feature double-coiled, heavy-gauge steel springs for increased tension capability and sturdiness. This makes the handgrips stronger, thus providing the user with a more strenuous workout. Handles are molded plastic with contoured fingergrips.

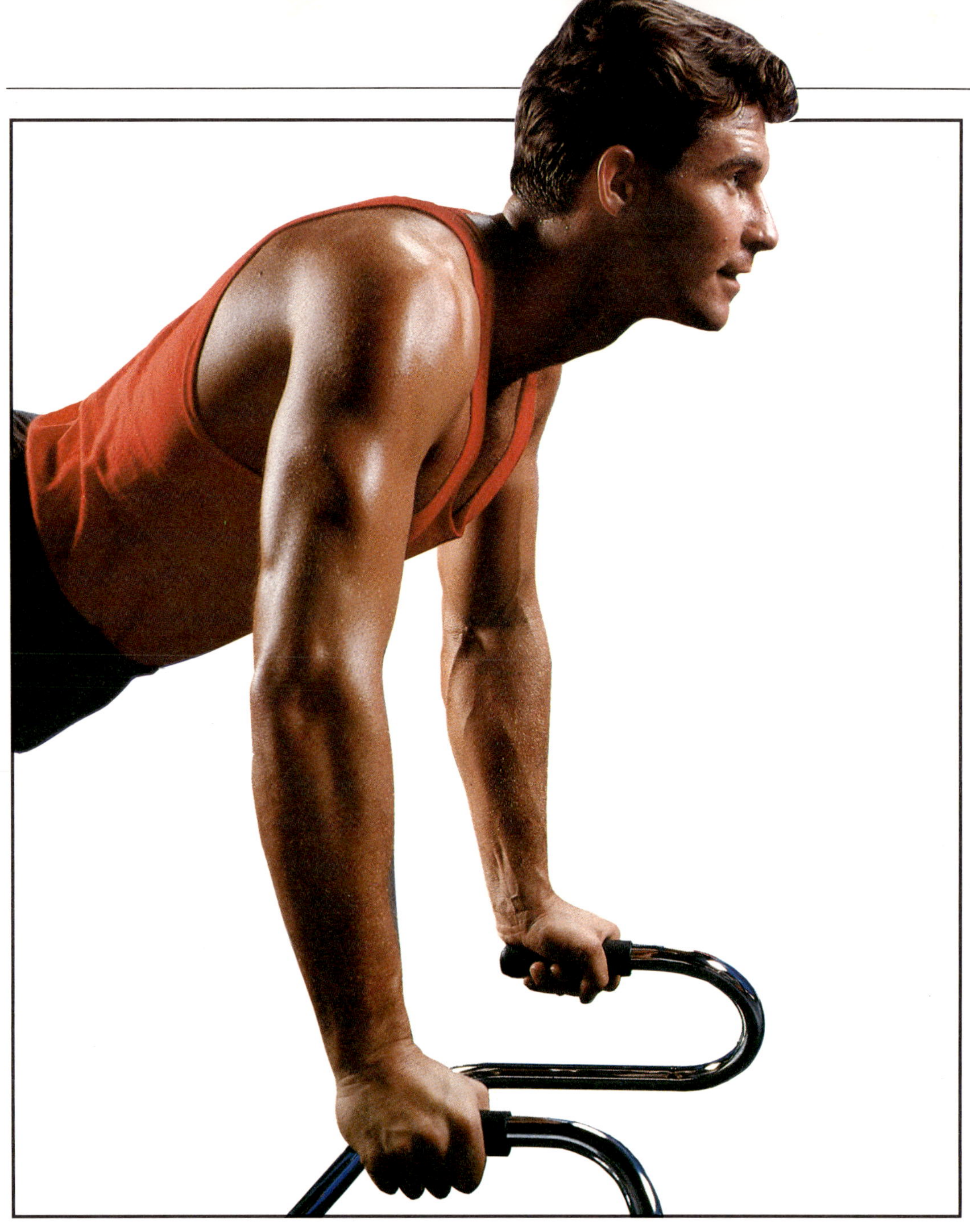

Avita Push-up Bar

Deep push-ups will stretch your pectoral muscles, build and tone your frontal deltoids, triceps, and the muscles of the lower back. They will also increase the flexion and extension of your upper-body muscles. Avita's Push-up Bar facilitates this by offering more stretching capacity than an ordinary push-up. The bar is made of chrome-plated steel tubing and features two cushioned foam rubber handgrips. It is 14 inches by 30 inches by 7 inches and weighs only 6 pounds (3 kilos).

AMF Jump Ropes

Jumping rope provides an excellent cardiovascular workout, especially when wearing wrist or ankle weights. Consistent use will increase physical endurance, improve coordination, and strengthen and tone leg and upper body muscles. Jump ropes are available in cotton or leather and are most commonly available in 8- or 9-foot lengths. The best ropes have a variety of wooden handles as well as chrome-plated spring joints with swivel action.

AMF has nine models of "skip" ropes available. The model 1R (shown here) is easy to handle, with just enough length at 8 feet 6 inches. They vary in materials used for handles, the rope itself, and fixture of handle to the rope. Ball-bearing attached handles provide best performance.

Kyga Stick

The Kyga Stick is an exercise bar with extraordinary flexibility: It can be used as a bodybuilding resistance machine, a jump rope, a free weight or a weightlifting device. Based on the idea that the body requires a full range of motion for uniform muscle development, a special Kygacise Program has been developed that incorporates a variety of routines in a continuous and gradual sequence.

The Kyga Stick, despite its name, is actually a complete exercise package. Finished in a special wrinkle-coat paint in black with chrome-plated end caps, the small and cleverly designed unit is based on a series of weighted cylinders which nest one inside the other. The Stick consists of two main cylinders, ten nested cylinders of varying weights, four end caps, one connector, an extender, and a rope. The connector serves to double the length and weight of the Kyga Stick or to vary the weight on each side, while the extender allows a broader separation of weights. With the extender in place, the Stick can be used for a variety of stretching and barbell exercises; when used in conjunction with the rope, the device will benefit the midsection and lower extremities. The total weight of the Stick can be varied from 3 to 21 pounds (1½ to 9½ kilos).

Dyna Bender

The Dyna Bender is a power exercise bar consisting of two chrome-plated steel tubes inserted into a tightly wound steel spring. Each end of the bar is fitted with a black pvc (polyvinyl chloride plastic) grip and nylon safety cord. Available in a variety of spring tensions, the Dyna Bender will develop your chest, back, neck, and arms.

A variety of exercises can be performed, but they all involve bending the spring by exerting pressure on the handgrips. The greater the angle deviated, the greater the power required to hold it. The Dyna Bender is made by Mattel.

AMF Exercise Rings

Formerly the exclusive domain of the professional gymnast, exercise rings have finally made their way into the home. Since their height is generally fixed at between 102 and 106 inches, a considerable amount of space is required for proper placement and usage.

AMF's exercise rings feature a three-part assembly: rings, straps, and cables. The tubular rings are molded fiberglass with an inside diameter of 180 millimeters (7 inches), ±1 millimeter. Individual nylon webbed straps are looped through rings allowing for slide and the flexibility required for the execution of your routine. The top of each strap clips into a loop at the end of nylon-coated cables, which attach to the ceiling. The entire system is tested to withstand 800 kilograms (1,760 pounds) and measures 3,000 millimeters (12 feet) from the bottom of the ring to the top of the cable.

Nu-Barre Portable Barre

The increasing popularity of warm-up exercises has taken the barre out of the dance studio and into the home. Most commonly used for balance and equilibrium in a dance or stretching routine, the versatility of these barres has been somewhat limited by the conventional stabilizing and connecting braces. These braces are the support system for the barre.

The development of the "total support" barre opened up the vital space beneath the barre, allowing a number of new stretching and strengthening exercises to be performed. More specifically, recommended usage is for static and semikinetic stretching of all body muscles before and after your activity in order to warm up and reduce muscular injury. A total workout for strengthening, however, is also possible by using your own body weight and gravity. Lifting all or part of your body weight above the barre (chin-ups, pull-ups, and dips) will develop and strengthen upper-body muscles in the arms, neck, chest, shoulders, and abdomen, as well as the upper and lower back muscles. Ideally, the barre will augment a regular conditioning program.

Nu-Barre Portable Barres are handcrafted with 1½-inch-diameter thin-wall steel tubing for both strength and portability. The barres all feature an exceptionally smooth finish made of an electrostatically applied epoxy-based powder, which is then baked. The result is an easy-to-clean, nonchip coating that will maintain its good looks indefinitely. Rubber tips are bolted into the barre's feet to prevent skidding and floor damage.

Nu-Barre's Touring models feature an innovative friction-lock mechanical connection that requires no tools to operate. One need only turn the thumbbolt to fasten or undo the components.

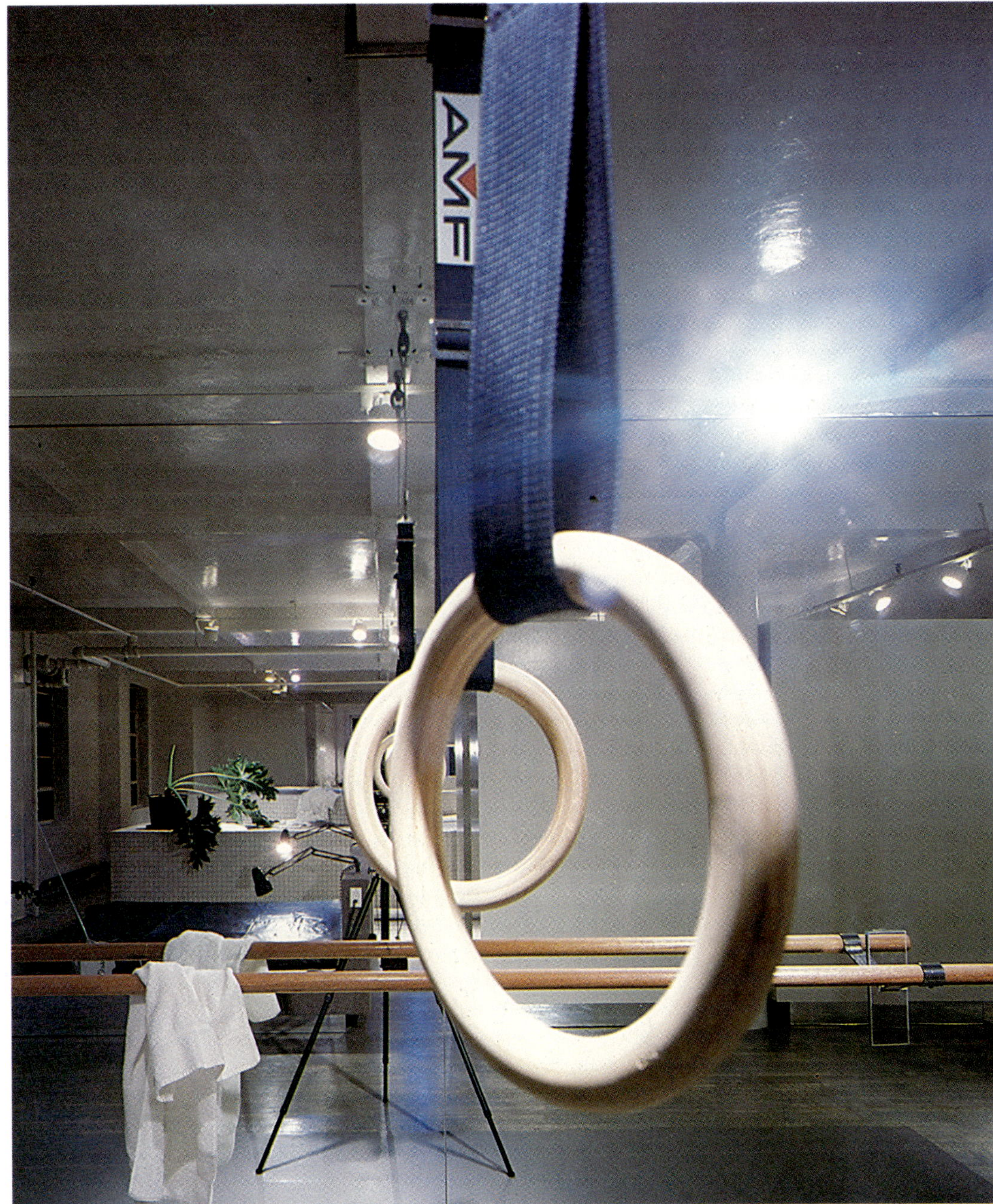

Adjustable nylon straps are looped through each of the tubular fiberglass rings allowing for maximum flexibility. A nylon-coated cable and clip assembly fastens each strap to the ceiling. The rings are generally set at between 102 and 106 inches above ground level.

ACCESSORIES

As technical breakthroughs become increasingly commonplace, it should come as no surprise to see electronics in step with the current fitness craze. No longer just frivolous playthings for the idle rich, the new electronic exercise accessories are serious training aids that chart the progress and efficiency of your workout. A mind-boggling array of processors, electrode sensors, and digital calculators now make cardiofitness measurement easier, more reliable, and more fun than ever before.

Some of the electronic aids highlighted in this chapter can track and record blood pressure, pulse rate, and body temperature; record distance, stride length, and step quantity when walking or jogging; read and display true EKG readings without tying you down—and there is even a talking scale to tell your weight via computer synthesized speech.

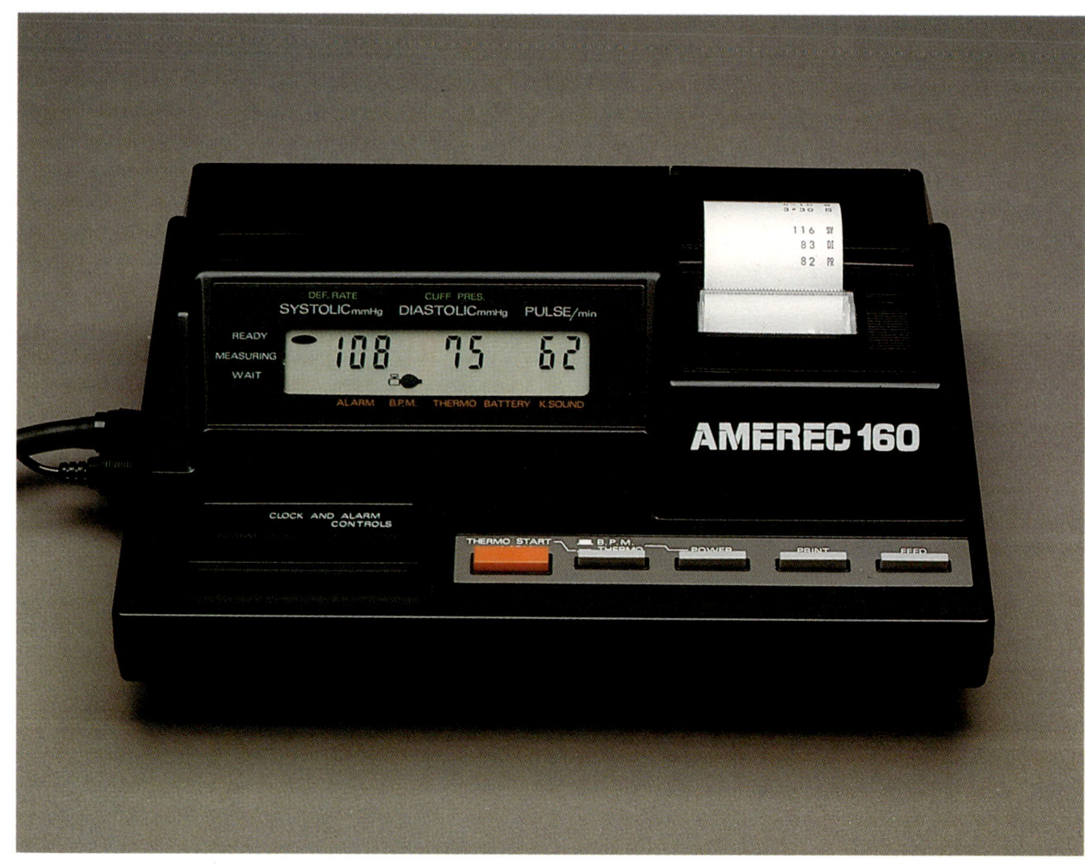

Amerec 160 Vital Signs Monitor

The Amerec 160 Vital Signs Monitor is a small, computerized tabletop unit for tracking and recording blood pressure, pulse rate, and body temperature. Vital signs are quickly measured and displayed on an easy-to-read LCD panel.

The 160 features high-tech styling, a matte black plastic housing, and measures only 9 x 6 x 2¾ inches. A narrow gray band sets off a fingertip control panel with five operational buttons. The horizontal LCD panel is obliquely angled for easy reading and is adjacent to the hard copy printer. A traditional inflation cuff (gray) features a Velcro closure, black cable connector, and squeeze bulb. A white thermoprobe records body temperature from under the tongue or armpit. There is also a built-in programmable reminder signal that can be set to alert you to take measurements at a particular time of day.

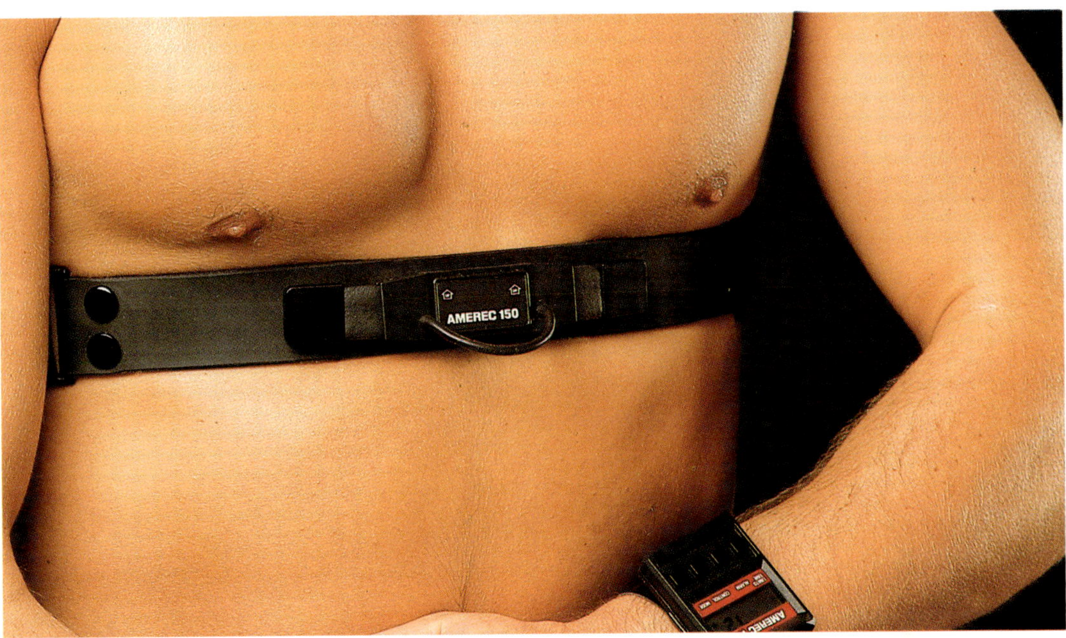

Cronus Pedometer

The Cronus Pedometer gives accurate readings for both walking and jogging. It fits neatly into the palm of your hand and features a matte black housing and three separate readouts: distance, stride length, and step quantity.

The distance jogged or walked automatically registers on the vertically calibrated scale (in miles or kilometers) mounted on the pedometer's top surface. Immediately adjacent, a graduated scale—color-coded to different stride lengths—shows total distance. The third scale is edge-mounted and shows a digital readout for the number of steps completed. The pedometer clips on one's belt or waistband and measures only 2 inches across and ½-inch thick.

Personal Sauna

The FITNESS Moist Sauna Model F310 offers the luxury of a home sauna without the inconvenience of structural or spatial modifications. Long used as a regular part of the post-exercise regimen, saunas promote relaxation, stimulate circulation, cleanse the skin and relieve minor aches and pains.

The Model F310 is a one-piece cast aluminum module which features a leak-proof door with no-lock safety mechanism and corrosion resistant hinge. Light-weight and portable (69 lbs) the Moist Sauna requires no special wiring or plumbing; for safety and accessibility, electrical controls are mounted on the outside of the cabinet. Additional conveniences include a built-in towel bar and adjustable seat and backrest.

Amerec 130 Pulsemeter

The Amerec 130 Pulsemeter is a training aid for monitoring pulse rate and elapsed time during an aerobic workout. When you attach the sensor clip (which is itself connected to the pulsimeter with a wire) to your earlobe, a tiny 4-bit microcomputer translates your heartbeats into pulse readouts on the LCD display panel. More versatile than the conventional pulsimeter, the 130 offers simultaneous readout of elapsed time and pulse rate. Its timekeeping function operates in two convenient modes: hour/minute or minute/second.

The Amerec 130 combines good design with advanced technology. Encased in a matte black plastic housing, it resembles a calculator, measuring only 4⅜ inches wide x 2¾ inches high x 1 inch deep. The LCD panel is placed along a horizontal axis for easy-to-read display; a small red stop/start button is placed in the lower right-hand corner. A mounting bracket expedites use with a stationary bike while a wrist strap and collar clip will secure the pulsimeter when jogging.

Amerec 150 Sport Tester Telemeter

The Amerec 150 Sport Tester Telemeter is a convenient heart rate monitor that displays true EKG readings without tying you down. Using advanced telemetry, which remotely transmits and receives your heart-rate data, it virtually eliminates the need of cables or cumbersome equipment to restrict your movement.

The Sport Tester Telemeter is actually two separate interdependent pieces of equipment: a transmitter and a receiver. The transmitter features an ABS plastic case in matte black and measures 3¼ x 1 x ½ inches. It is affixed to the exterior surface of an adjustable, beltlike chest harness. By attaching the belt firmly around your chest just below the breast bone, the transmitter is able to pick up your heart rate from its source and send it to the receiver. The receiver is housed in a small matte black ABS plastic case. It features a 6-digit LED display and measures 2¼ x 1 x ½ inches. Four buttons control the clock mode, stopwatch function, heart-rate mode, and memory mode. The receiver can either be attached to the perforated wrist strap (it looks like a digital watch) or slipped into the harness holder.

Datatrim Talking Scale

To add zest to your weigh-in, try Datatrim's Talking Scale which will actually tell you your weight via computer-synthesized speech as you step on to the vinyl-covered platform. But Datatrim does not stop there—it will also help you stick to your diet by making appropriate comments!

After programming your diet goal into the scale (which can monitor two different people simultaneously), Datatrim will tell you your present weight and make encouraging comments on your daily progress or lack of it. The scale's waist-level control panel displays weight, the date, goal weight, and the number of days it will take to reach it.

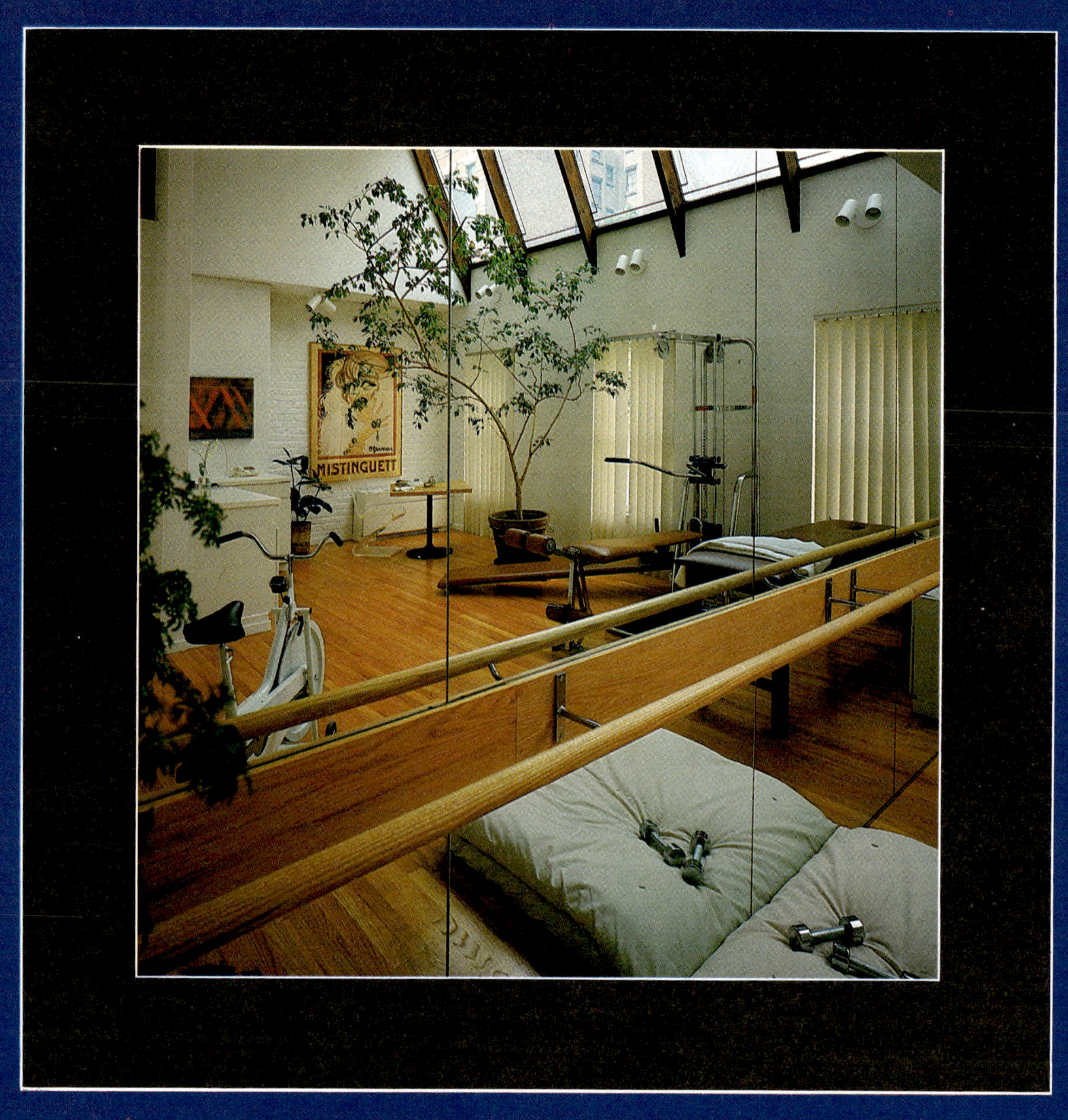
MISTINGUETT

CHAPTER TWO

DESIGN PORTFOLIO

New and perhaps unfamiliar ingredients must be considered when planning your home gymnasium. For example, your ceiling must be of sufficient height and your floor strong enough to support the size and extra weight of some of the equipment you may be considering. The space should comfortably accommodate the equipment while still enabling traffic to flow steadily and without interruption. Machines must follow a reasonable workout flow. Materials throughout should be durable, easily-cleaned, and odor-resistant. Wet, semi-wet, and dry areas must be sufficiently separate and properly ordered; ventilation must, at the very least, be adequate. What remains, then, is to establish that elusive point of intersection between functional and aesthetic compatibility.

The following Design Portfolio might just help. By showcasing home gymnasiums belonging to, among others, fitness enthusiasts, film stars, and professional athletes, this chapter offers a design palette ranging from the sublime to the outlandish. Use as many of their ideas as you want—in combination with your own—to create your own personal statement of fitness and style.

—Photographs by Dan Eifert

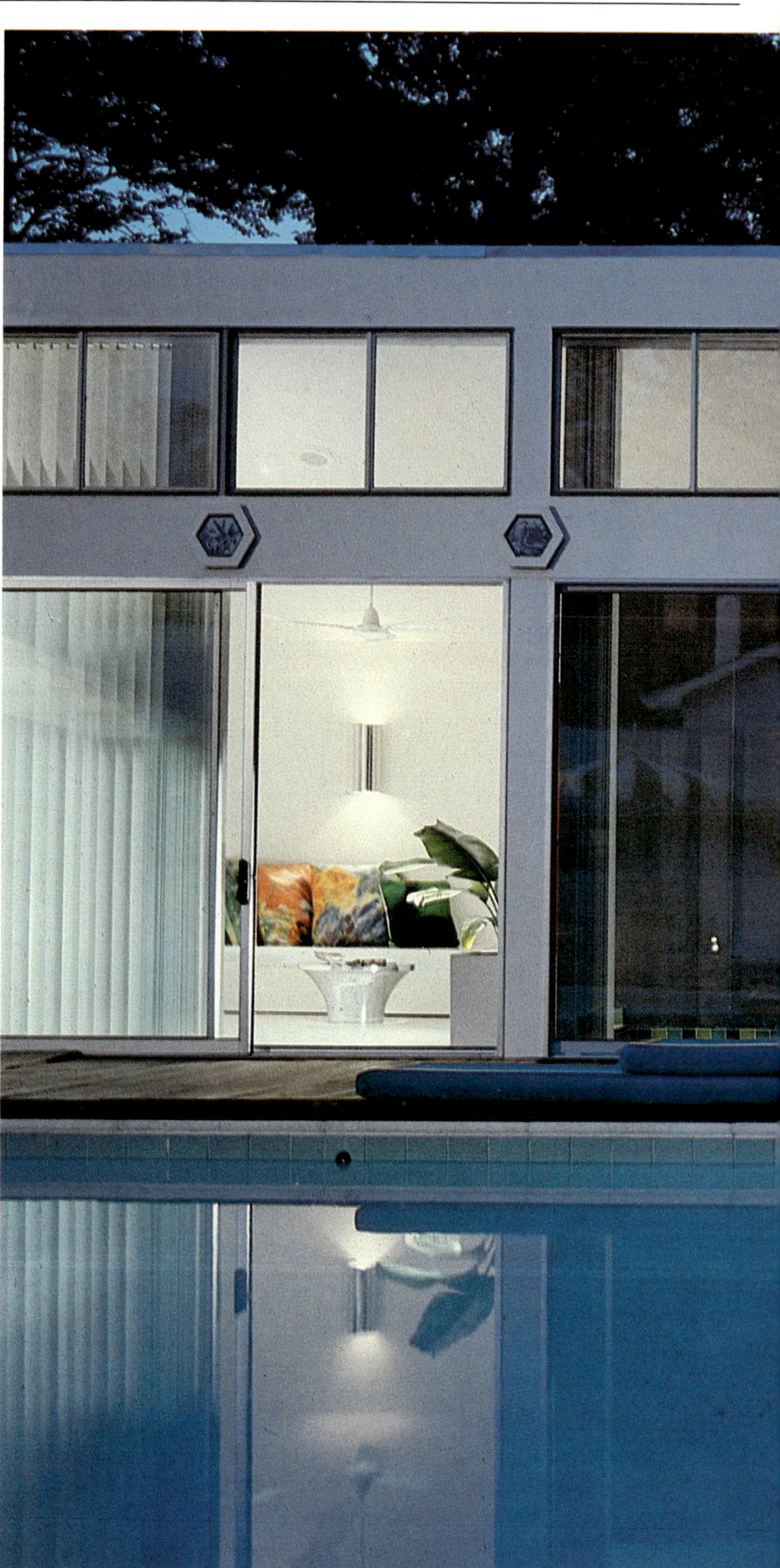

POOLSIDE LUXURY

For this Southampton, New York, estate, designer Rubén De Saavedra created a sybaritic health club and home gymnasium. Seeing to every amenity, Mr. De Saavedra designed a suite of rooms, each with its own functional identity. Set along the swimming pool's horizontal axis, in its own physical fitness wing, a tiled soak-tub is flanked by the gymnasium on one side and a lounge on the other. An oversized whirlpool and adjoining dressing room are situated out of sight, behind the soak-tub's tiled partition wall.

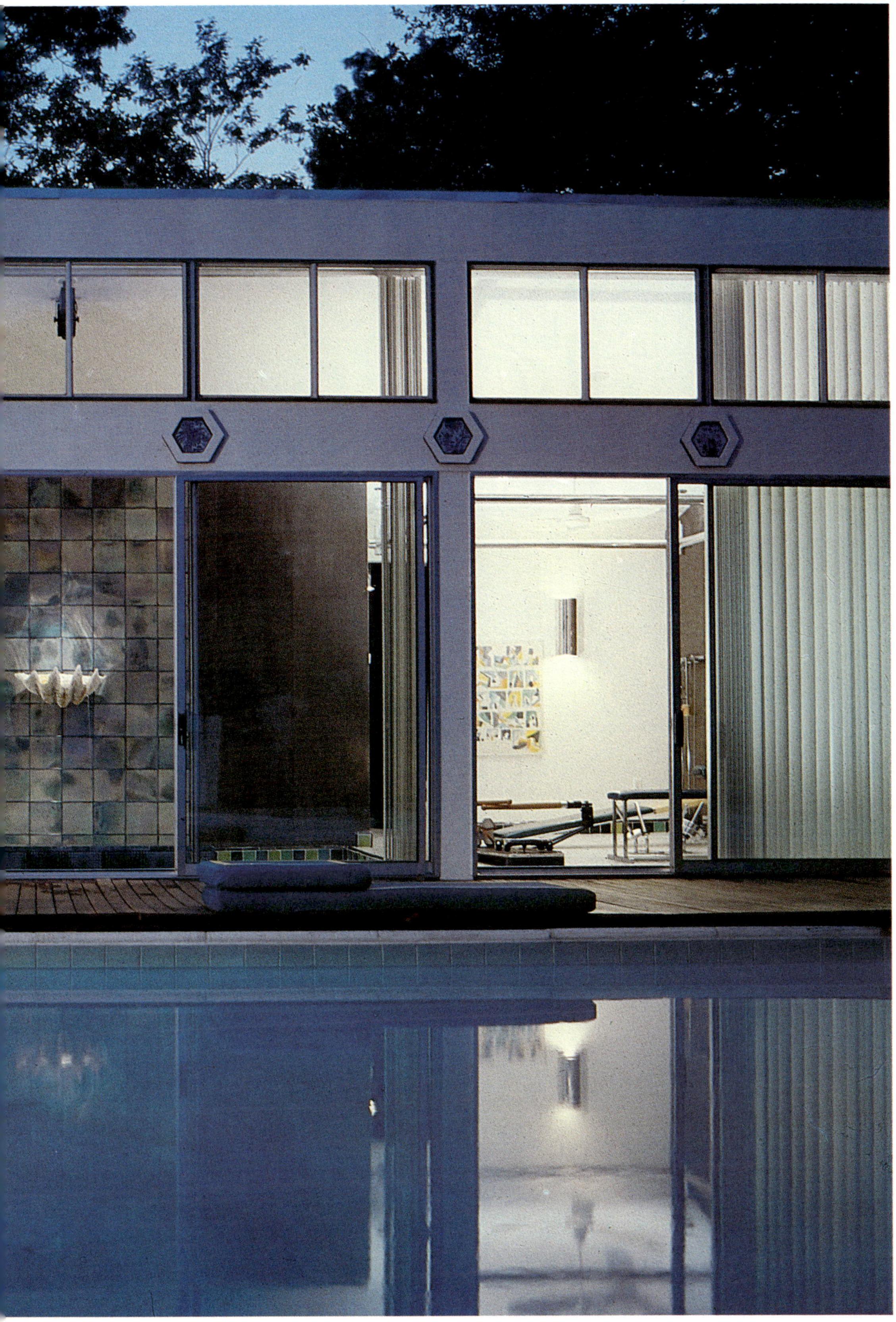

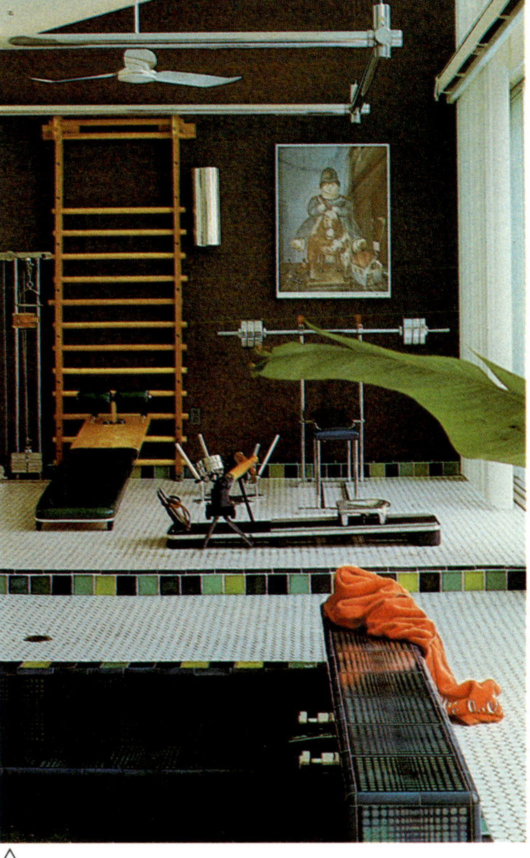

△ To relieve its Spartan austerity, Mr. De Saavedra specified a bittersweet chocolate wall adorned with a single painting from the client's collection. Functionally, the gym is equipped with a wall-mounted multiuse gym, free weights, abdominal board with ankle rollers, and slant board with minitrainer (wall ladder). The ceiling fan ensures a comfortable workout.

◁ The poolside location of this health club/gymnasium is enhanced by sliding glass doors and a clerestory. The tiled partition wall, at center, backs a sunken tub and open shower. A large clamshell wall sconce adds a resonant touch of nautical fantasy. The tub is flanked by the gym on the right and by the lounge on the left.

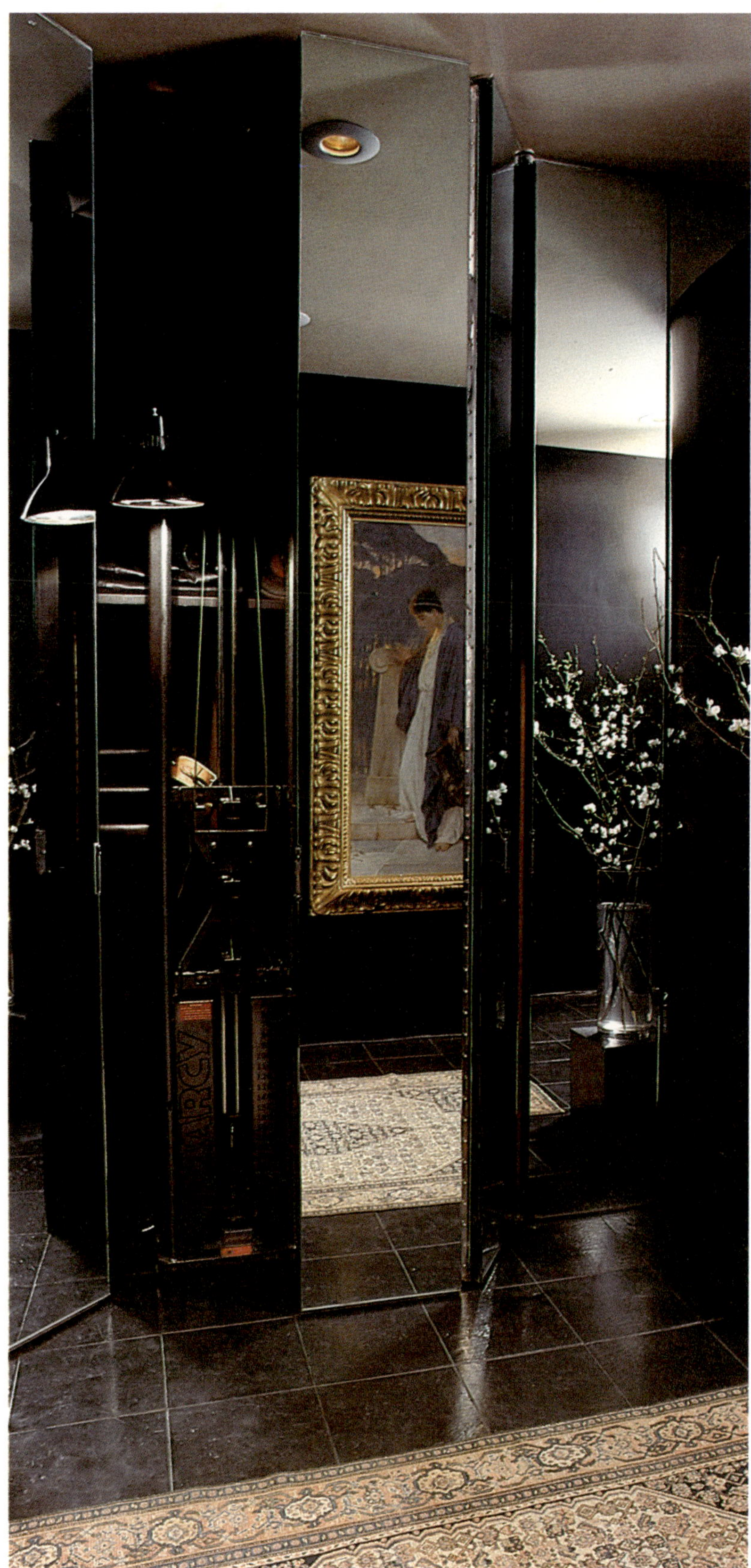

Mirror-clad bi-fold doors conceal a Marcy weightlifting machine; exercise mat and dumbbells are stored on an overhead shelf. A turn-of-the-century painting by Alma-Tadema and an antique Persian carpet counterpoint the all-black color palette.

URBAN INGENUITY

For this townhouse gymnasium, designer Eric Bernard demonstrates his own very special brand of sophisticated ingenuity. Tucked into a foyer closet behind mirror-clad bi-fold doors is a complete home-fitness center. As a glamorous anteroom for receiving guests, the foyer's identity is easily transformed by opening the closet doors and setting the supine bench and exercise mat in place. A master of surface detail, Bernard has carefully orchestrated mirror, tile, and sculpted wall forms to enliven the all-black color palette with textural interest. A turn-of-the-century painting by Alma-Tadema and an antique Persian carpet lend a traditional note.

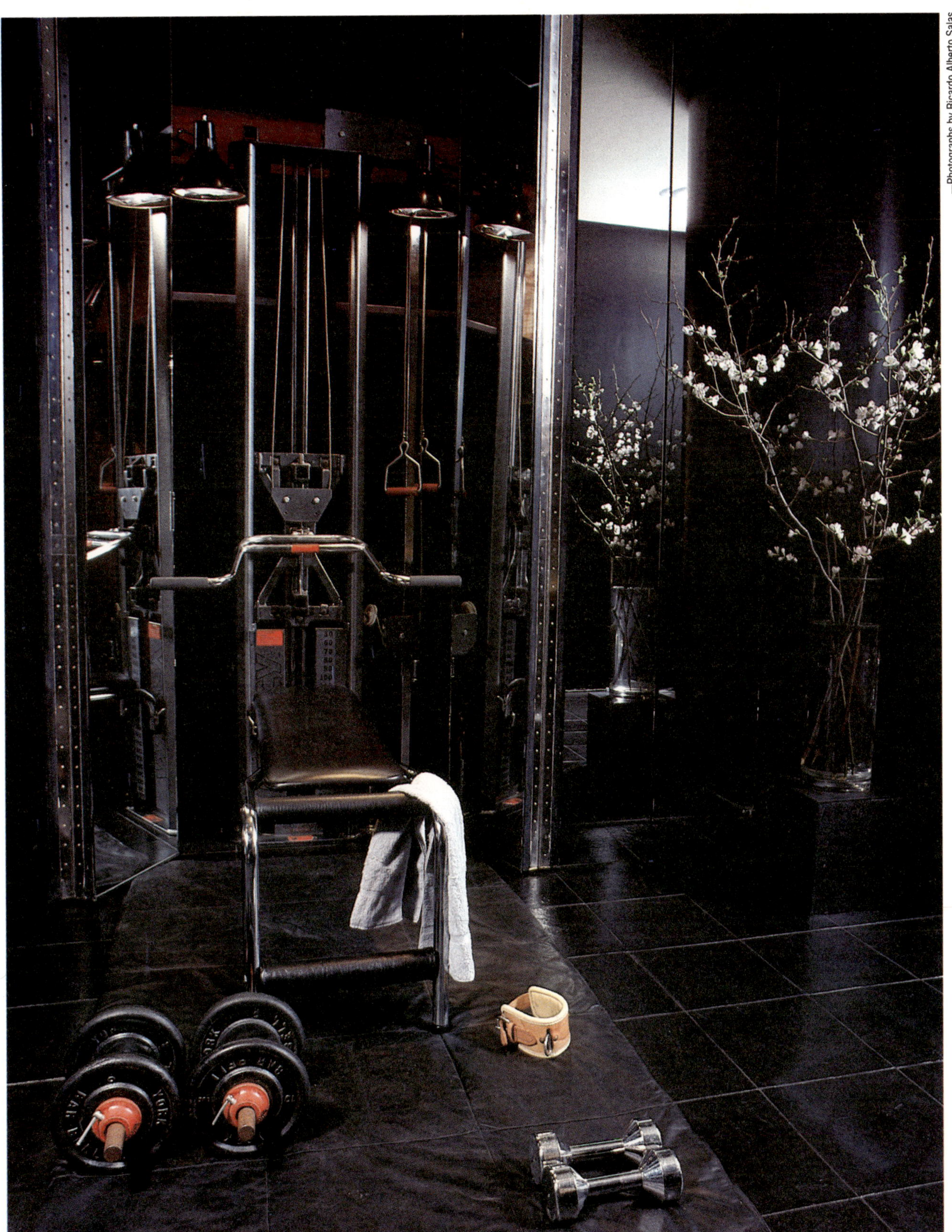

—Photographs by Ricardo Alberto Salas

With the detachable incline bench and exercise mat in place, the foyer is easily transformed into a complete home-fitness center. A simple crystal vase with flowering branches recalls the Japanese art of ikebana.

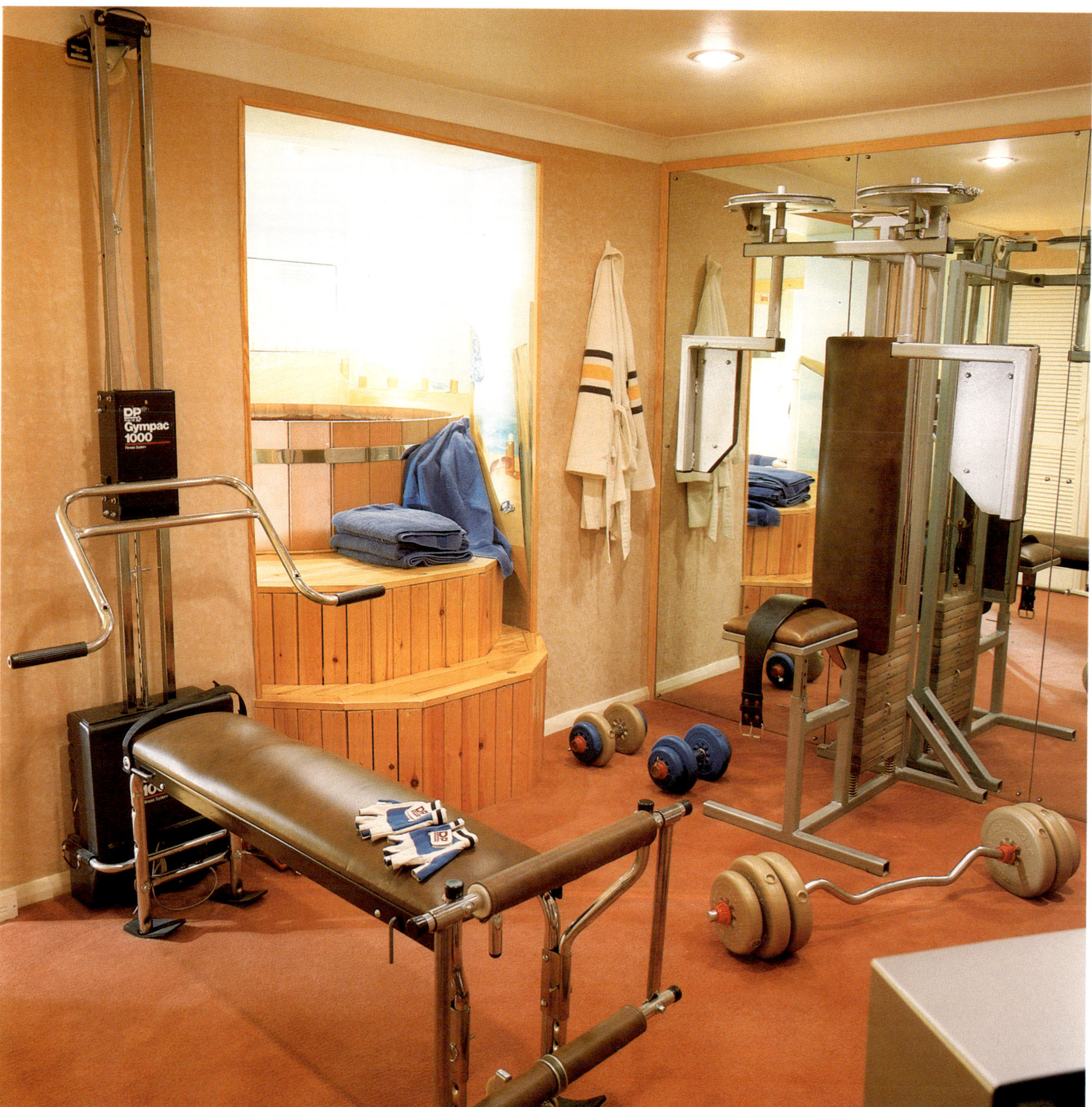

—Photographs by Jerry Tubby/EWA

The hot tub is supported by a tiered platform covered in vertical pine planking. The chrome-plated weightlifting machine and Nautilus station feature leather-covered contact surfaces; a mirrored wall amplifies the windowless space.

A trompe l'oeil seaside mural enlivens the windowless niche around the hot tub. The painted door with ventilating grill leads to a sauna; ceiling-mounted floodlights are dimmer-controlled for ambient effect.

SEASIDE HOT TUB

A complete home-fitness center with central hot tub—this was the commission proposed to the interior designer by his clients. In what was to become the mainstay of the entire gym, the designer's solution was to raise the tub on a double height platform and set it inside its own niche. As an added bonus the walls of the enclosure were treated with a trompe l'oeil mural offering a lively view of the seashore replete with cabanas and bulkhead moorings. Raising the tub as shown also eliminated the more costly plumbing and drainage plan that a floor-mounted solution would have required.

Training equipment is arranged around the tub enclosure and includes a wall-mounted DP 2000 Gympac as well as a curl bar and dumbbells, both fitted with plastic-coated weight plates. Coloration of the space intentionally mitigates the notion of home gymnasiums as high-tech command posts—walls are a flattering peach color while the floor treatment is an unexpectedly luxurious velvet pile carpeting in a slightly darker shade. A television monitor and videocassette recorder were installed to screen the clients' exercise tapes.

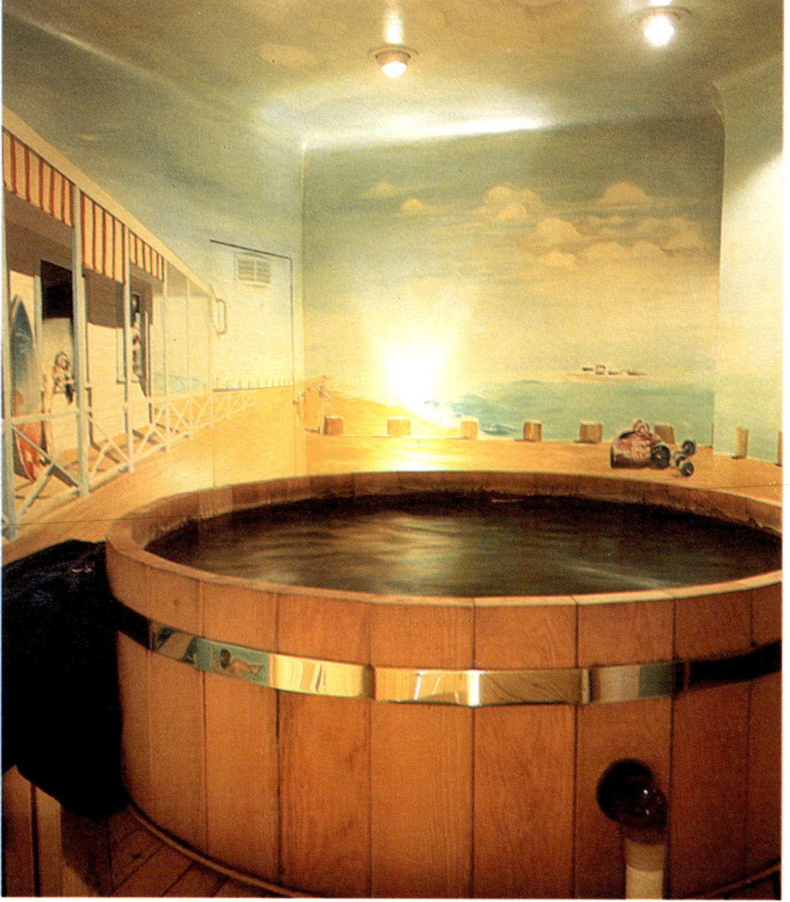

A truncated partition defines this mezzanine-level gymnasium located in a spacious loft. Postmodern colors, wood accents, and glass clerestories soften the architectural programme.

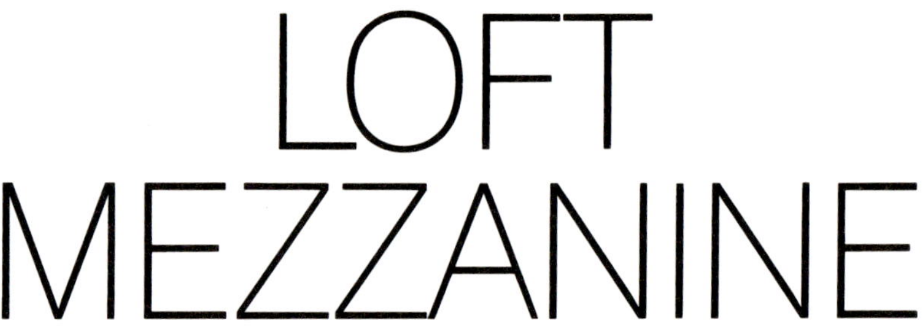

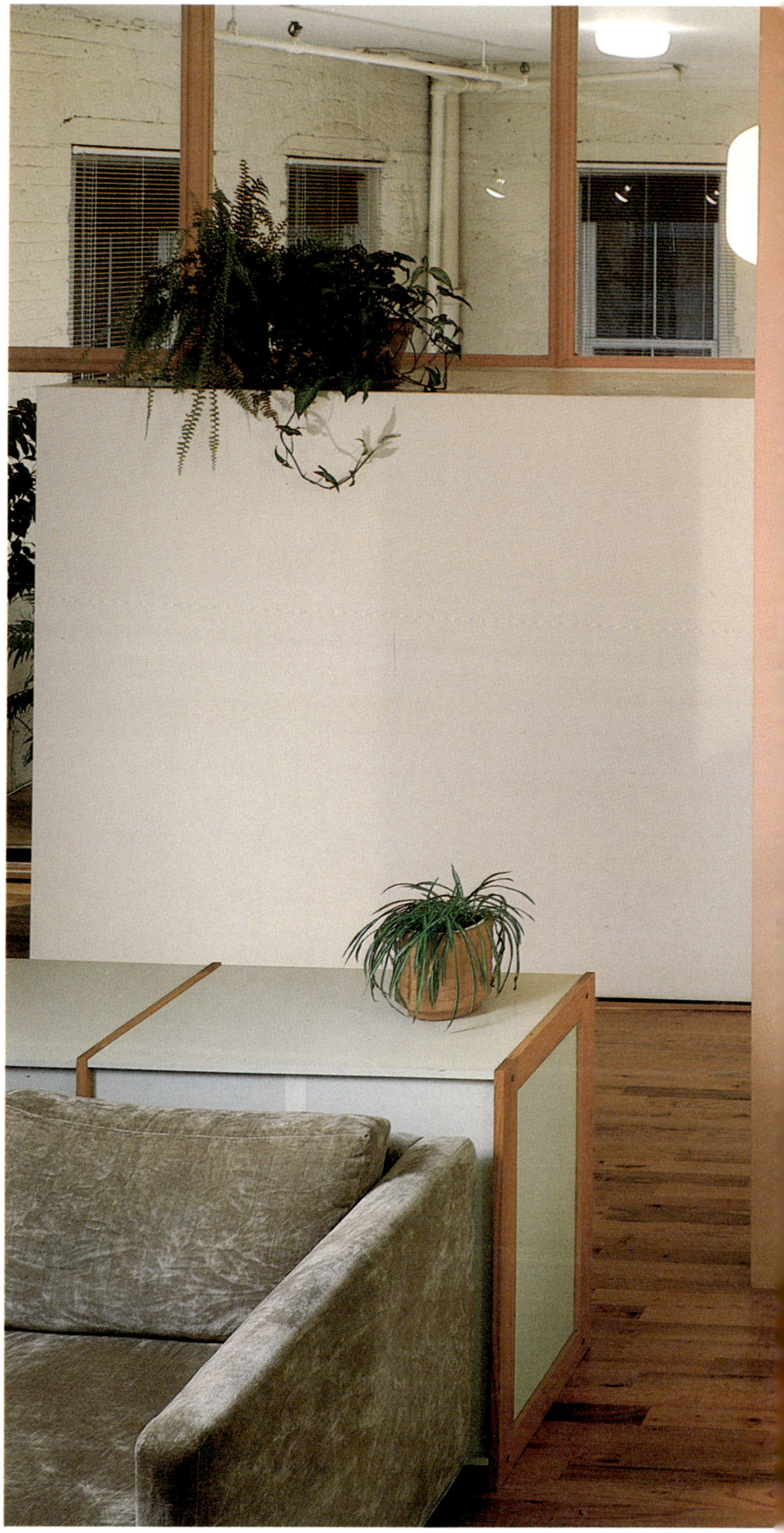

LOFT MEZZANINE

Loft spaces offer unbridled creative opportunities seldom encountered in urban design commissions. This loft, designed by architect Chris Chimera, is no exception. Rather than a vast undifferentiated space, Chimera used partitions, columns, and clerestories to define a series of interrelated functional enclaves. A postmodern color palette of muted pink and seafoam green enhances the architectural elements and softens the austerity of the otherwise all-white space.

A white, curved pipe railing defines the access stairway leading to the mezzanine-level gymnasium. Bound by a truncated partition and clerestory, this compact workout zone enjoys privacy without isolation. Exercise mats and dumbbells share the space with a complete selection of weight training equipment, a dancer's barre, and a stationary bicycle. The floor is covered with industrial grade carpeting laid over double-thick foam padding.

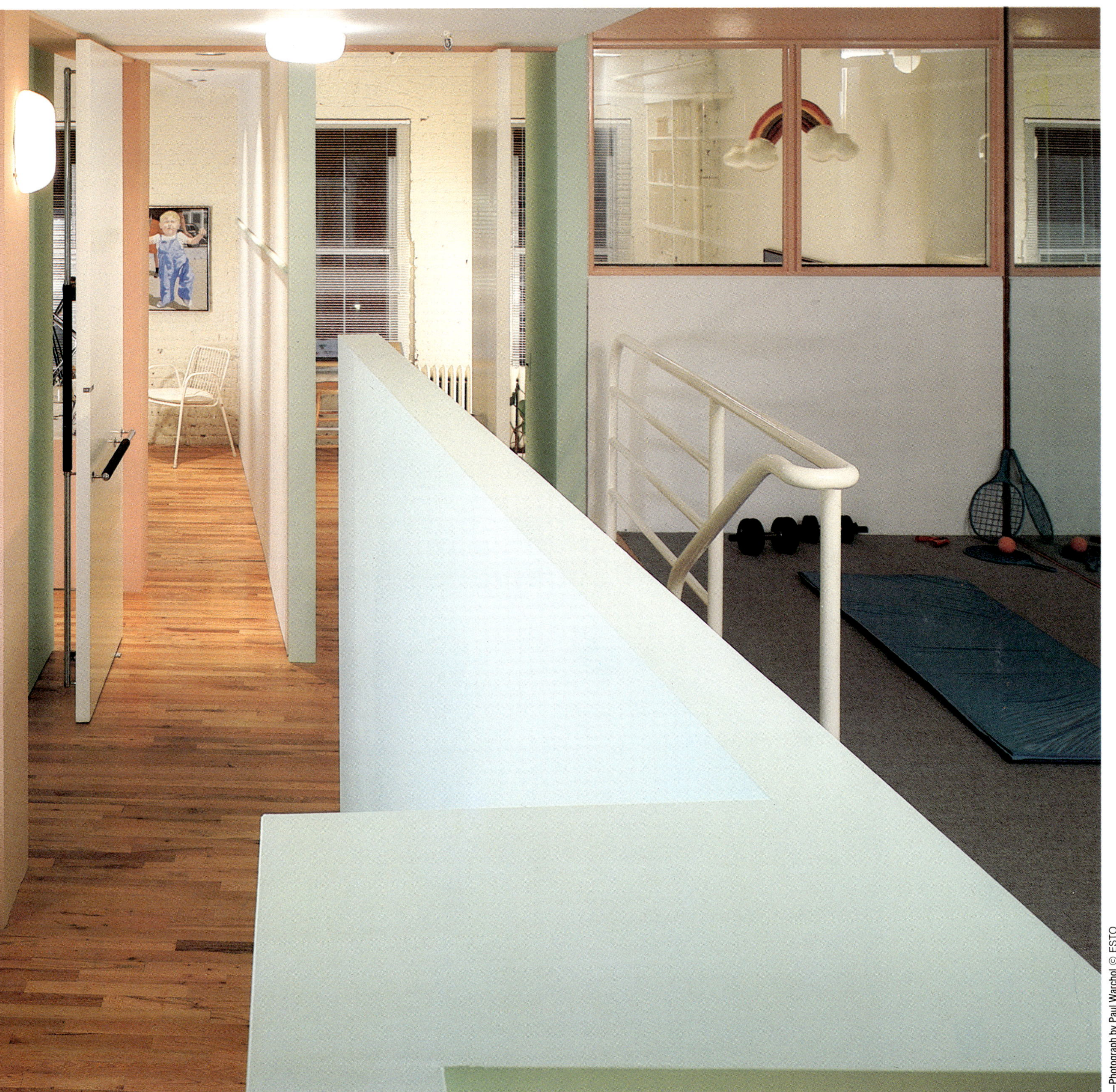

—Photograph by Paul Warchol © ESTO

Designer Kirk sets the newest electronic equipment against a traditional background. An existing *bibliothèque* now holds towels, dumbbells, and treasured memorabilia. The hanging milk glass and brass oil lamp are nineteenth-century Dutch Nouveau.

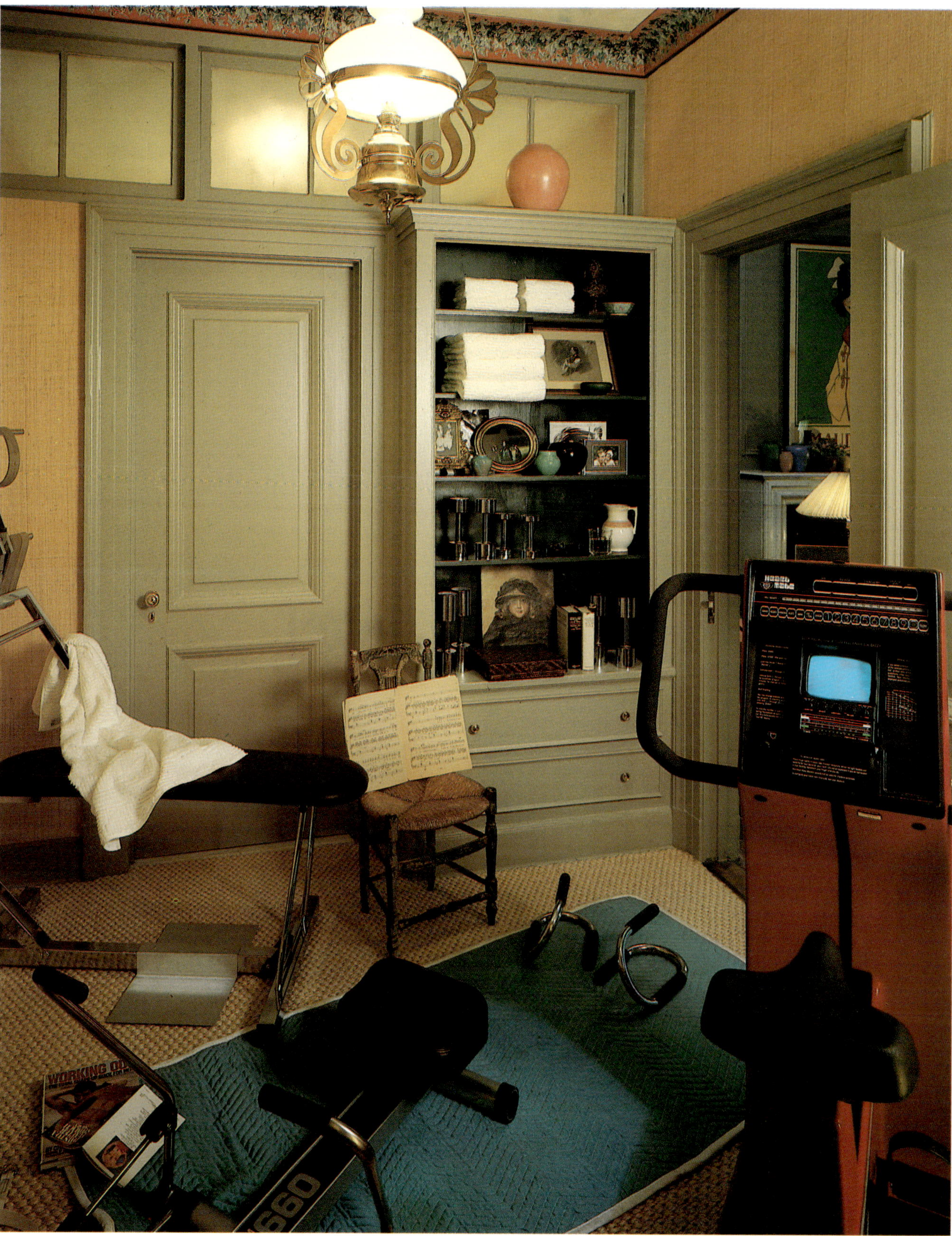

—Photographs by Michael Dunne/EWA

Warm colors in the glazed chintz slipcovers and Indian-pattern rugs enhance the cozy feeling of the music room. Displayed on the mantel is a collection of vibrantly colored twentieth-century American pottery; between the windows, a nineteenth-century American Empire *faux bois* chest. ▷

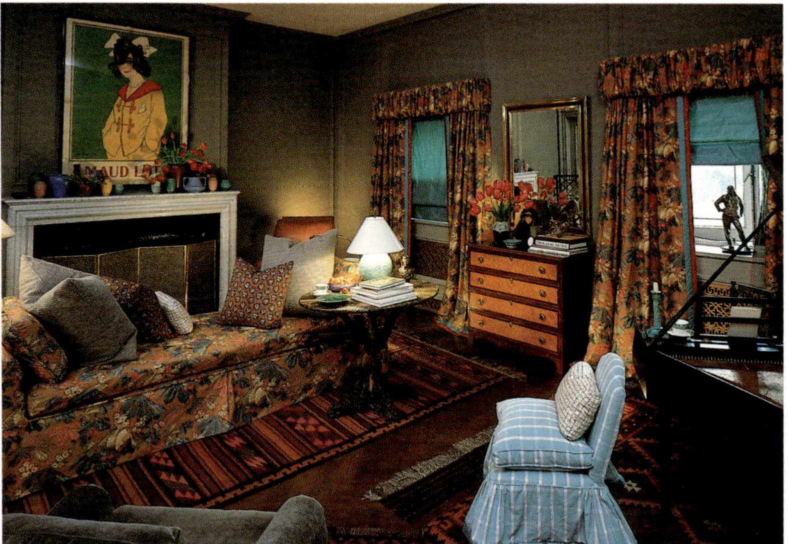

One of the music room's focal points, the harpsichord features a trompe l'oeil, fantasy finish by painter Mark West. ▽

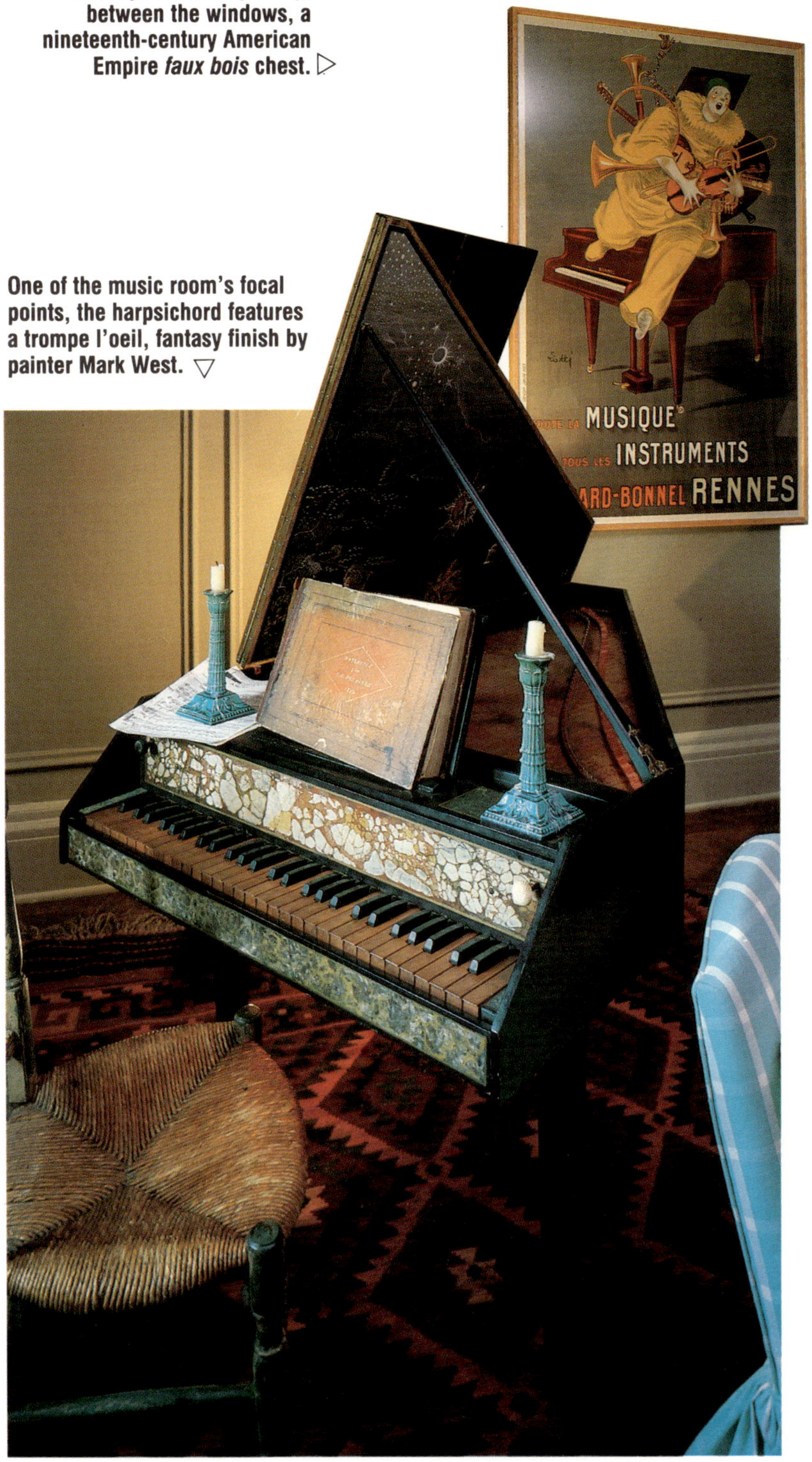

BAROQUE TECH

For clients whose passions run from baroque music to physical fitness, designer Carey Kirk created a special entertainment suite on the top level of their New York townhouse. Instead of structural modifications, designer Kirk enhanced the existing architectural character with a palette of elegant surface treatments and furnishings.

In the music room, a melange of eighteenth- and nineteenth-century furnishings and accessories have been integrated to give a warm, inviting look. An overscaled daybed provides numerous seating possibilities alone or in conjunction with a velvet club chair and slipcovered side chair. The curtains repeat the daybed fabric and set off the light blue Roman shades. Replete with trompe l'oeil harpsichord (painted by Mark West), the music room has been used for a full range of social events from soirées to cocktail parties.

Crowned with a fantasy all its own, the small gymnasium features a trompe l'oeil cloud-filled sky, also painted by Mark West. A fine-woven sisal mat on the wall is complemented by a sisal mat of much heavier gauge as a floor treatment. An impressive equipment profile includes a Heart Mate stationary ergometer equipped with color television, AM/FM radio, and electronic fitness test control panel; Amerec 660 Rowing Machine; and Space Gym with supine bench and Olympic Bars. Kirk fitted an existing *étagère* with glass shelves for storage of a chrome-plated dumbbell set, towels, and assorted memorabilia. A quilted movers mat is used for floor exercises.

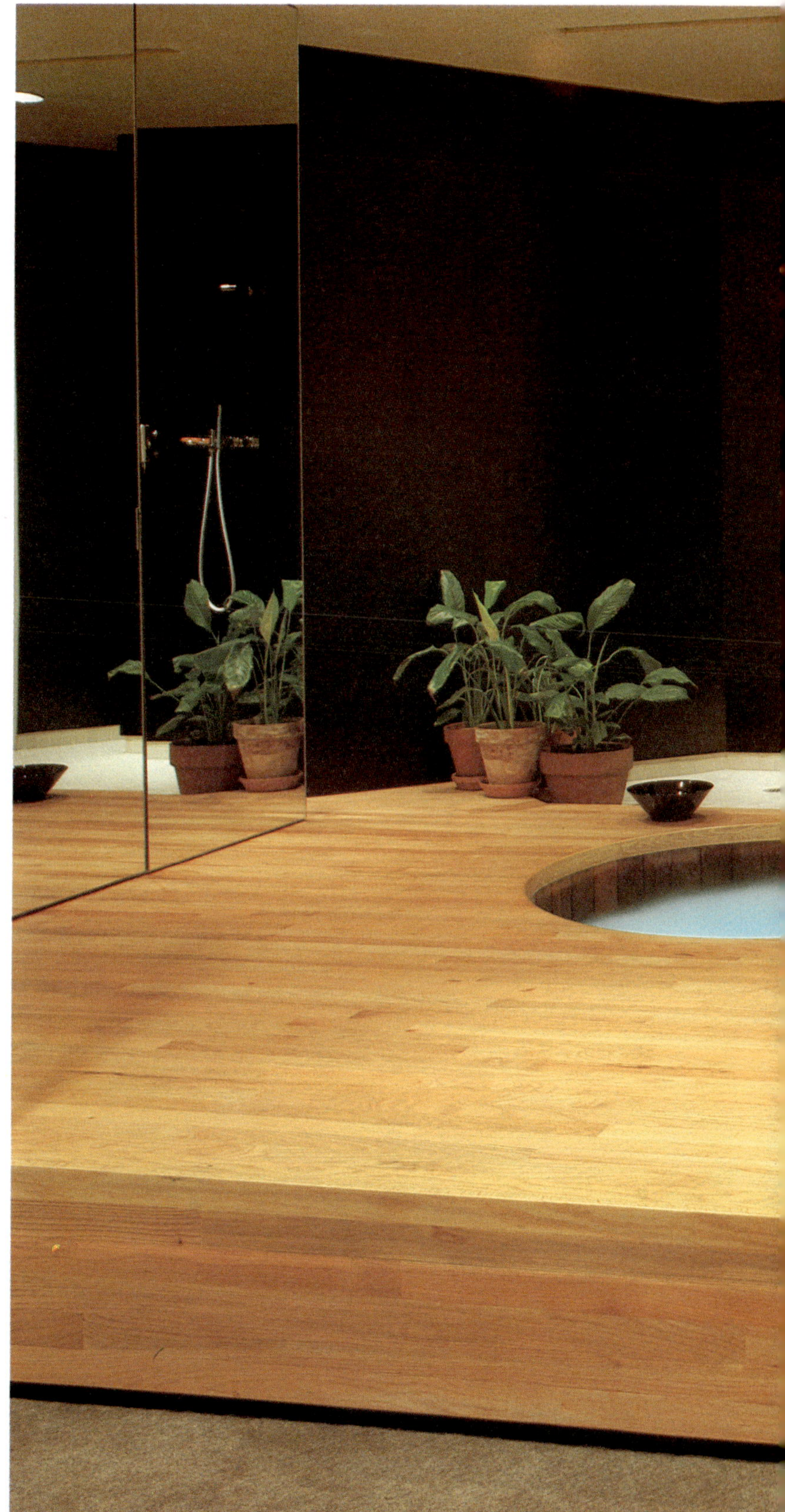

ARTISTIC EXPRESSION

For an artist, the joy of his work lies not only in its design but in its execution. Sculptor/designer Robert Mihalik realized this satisfaction by not only designing his own fitness center but constructing it as well. With an eye for spatial integrity, Mihalik recalls the Japanese approach to design. Texture and materials are varied according to functional compatibility: polyurethaned oak around the hot tub, carpeting for weight work, and leather-covered mat for floor exercises.

Located in Mihalik's spacious Soho loft, the space shown here also functions as the designer's bedroom—with its black leather cover, the sleeping futon doubles as an exercise mat. Practical considerations notwithstanding, Mihalik uses floor-to-ceiling panels for functional and spatial compatibility. The white panels beside the tub, for example, conceal voluminous storage space, a library, and a fully-equipped audio/video station. Water closet amenities are located across the oak platform where an open mirror panel reveals a black laminate-clad shower with Aarne Jacobsen designed fittings. Mirror panels can be closed to effectively hide the area from view.

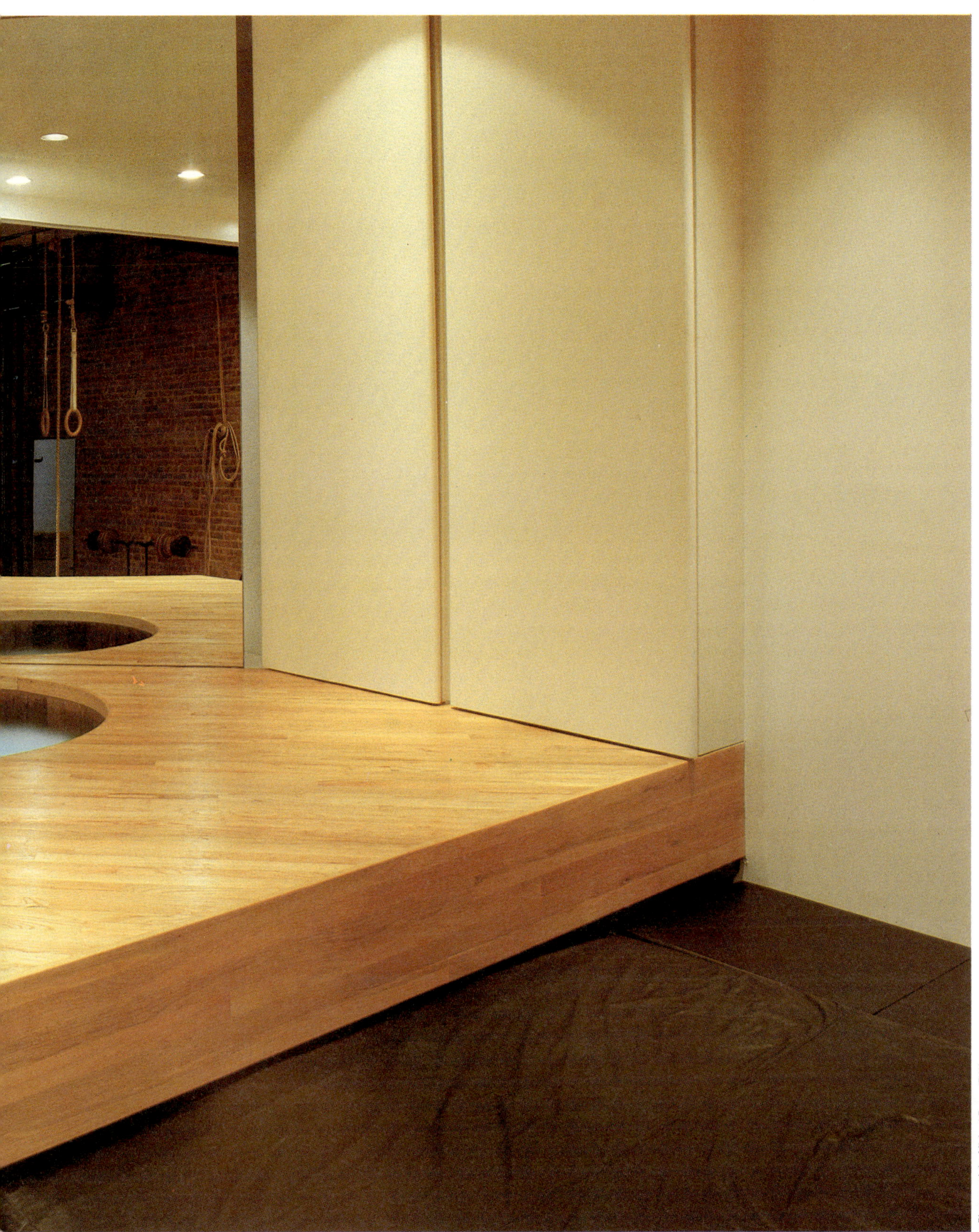

—Photograph by Michael Dunne/EWA

A circular soak-tub takes center stage atop an oblique-angled oak platform. The black laminate-clad shower is visible beyond the tub; the black leather-covered futon doubles as an exercise mat.

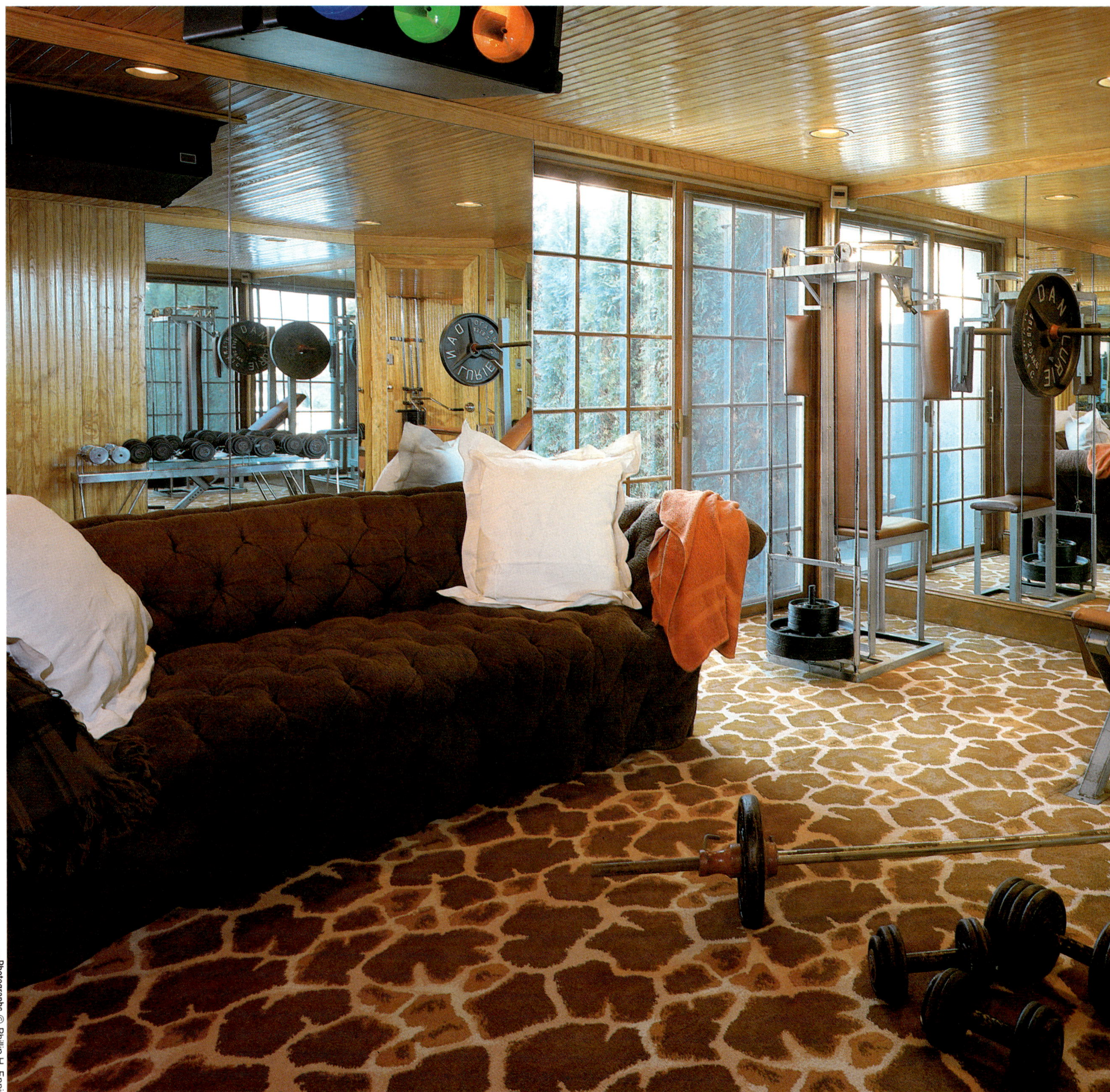

—Photographs © Phillip H. Ennis

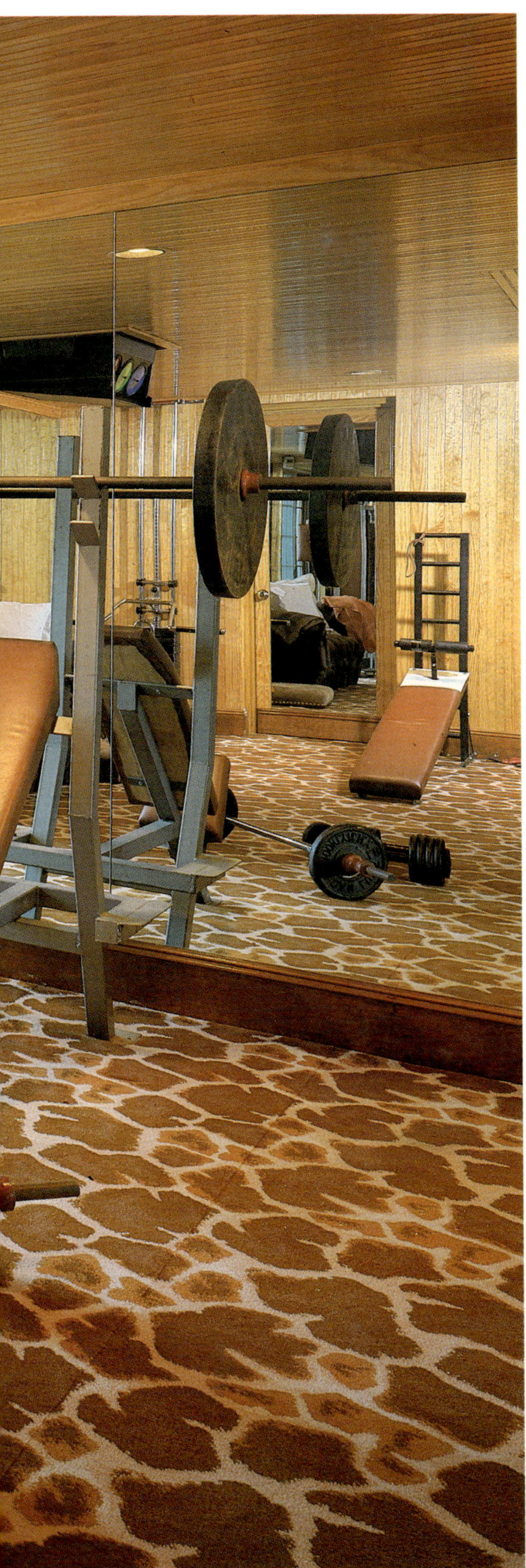

◁ **A paneled wall and ceiling treatment adds warmth and subtle visual interest to this entertainment suite. The tufted suede sofa is perfect for relaxing or watching the large-screen television by means of the overhead projector. The carpet's animallike motif lends a note of jungle exotica.**

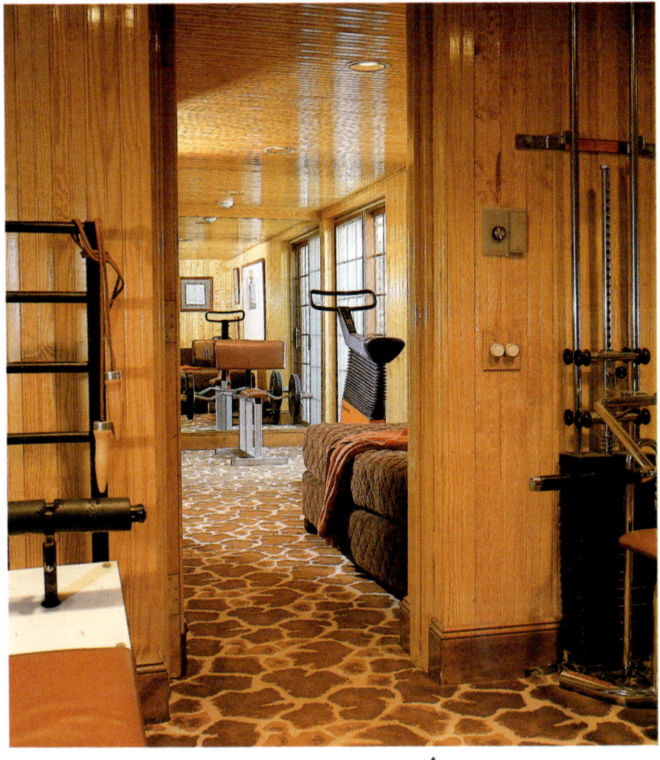

△ **A multistation weightlifting machine and slant board flank the entrance to the guest room. To accommodate postexercise relaxation, the bed is dressed in diamond-quilted suede; mirror panels along the back wall reflect an electronic Lifecycle and weightlifting bench.**

VARIETAL VINTAGE

One of the more difficult challenges in interior design is meeting the joint demands of function and elegance. When, in addition to these, the call is for a country home, the need for careful editing is even greater. Designers Robert Denning and Vincent Fourcade have addressed the problem with characteristic spirit and a touch of the unexpected.

Located in a fashionable New York vacation resort, this home gymnasium/guest suite is as much a comment on design as it is an eloquent projection of the owner's personality. Against a backdrop of paneled walls, animal-pattern carpeting, and tufted Chesterfield sofa, a selection of exercise equipment takes a brutal yet compatible stance. Presiding over the entire room, a ceiling-mounted television projector accommodates the luxury of large-screen entertainment. The genius of this space lies in its adaptability—all is planned with the aim of allowing the client to orchestrate the visual and social experiences within. Seen from this point of view, the entertainment suite is paradigmatic in its blend of fine materials and European approach to living.

An incline bench and barbells assume considerable design significance as part of this living room vignette. Black-lacquer spheroid from Luther Antiques; leather hide from Jay Quintana.

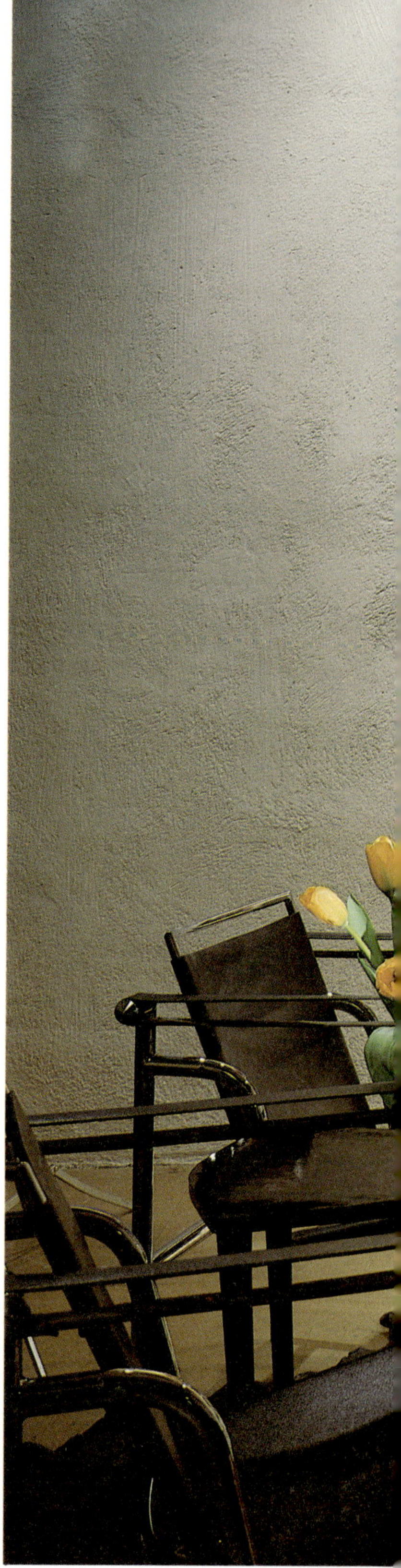

ARTFUL VIGNETTE

With an eye for the theatrical, New York-based designer James Franklin Mitchell created this unusual vignette for client Jay Quintana. Successfully commingling the classic and the experimental, Mitchell combines vintage chairs, contemporary art, and high-tech exercise equipment with freewheeling confidence and spirit.

The outcome of this vignette was as much the result of spatial considerations as of an understanding client. Rather than devote precious space to an exclusive activity, Mitchell boldly liberated the concept of home fitness by introducing the actual equipment as a component design element in the living area. Sharing space with barbells and an incline bench are Le Corbusier's version of the traditional British officer's chair—which he designed in collaboration with Charlotte Perriand in 1928—and a 1950s-style lacquer cigarette table of questionable pedigree. Under the watchful eye of an anonymous painting, a black-lacquer spheroid and leather hide (on the floor) complete the setting.

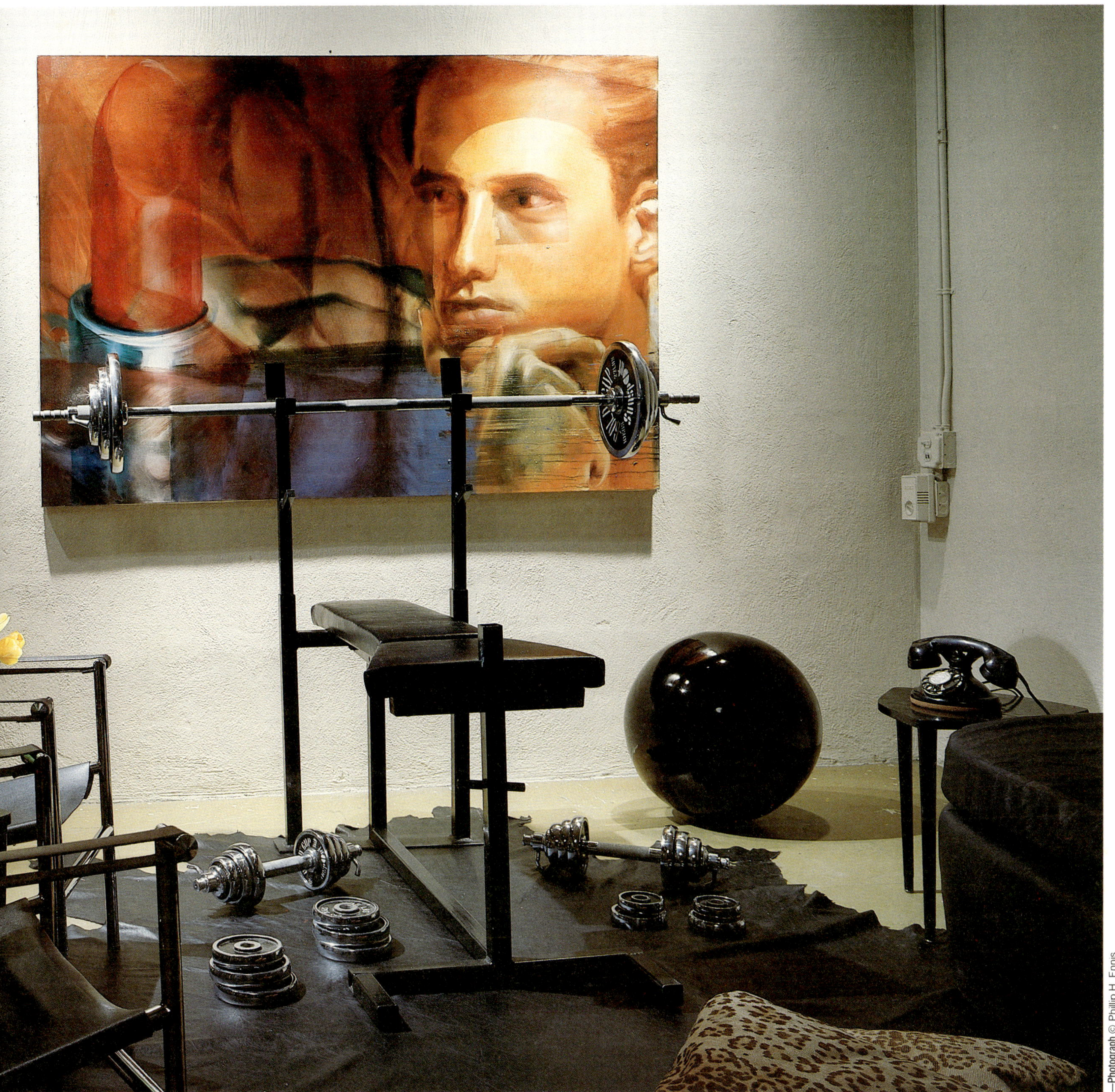

—Photograph © Phillip H. Ennis

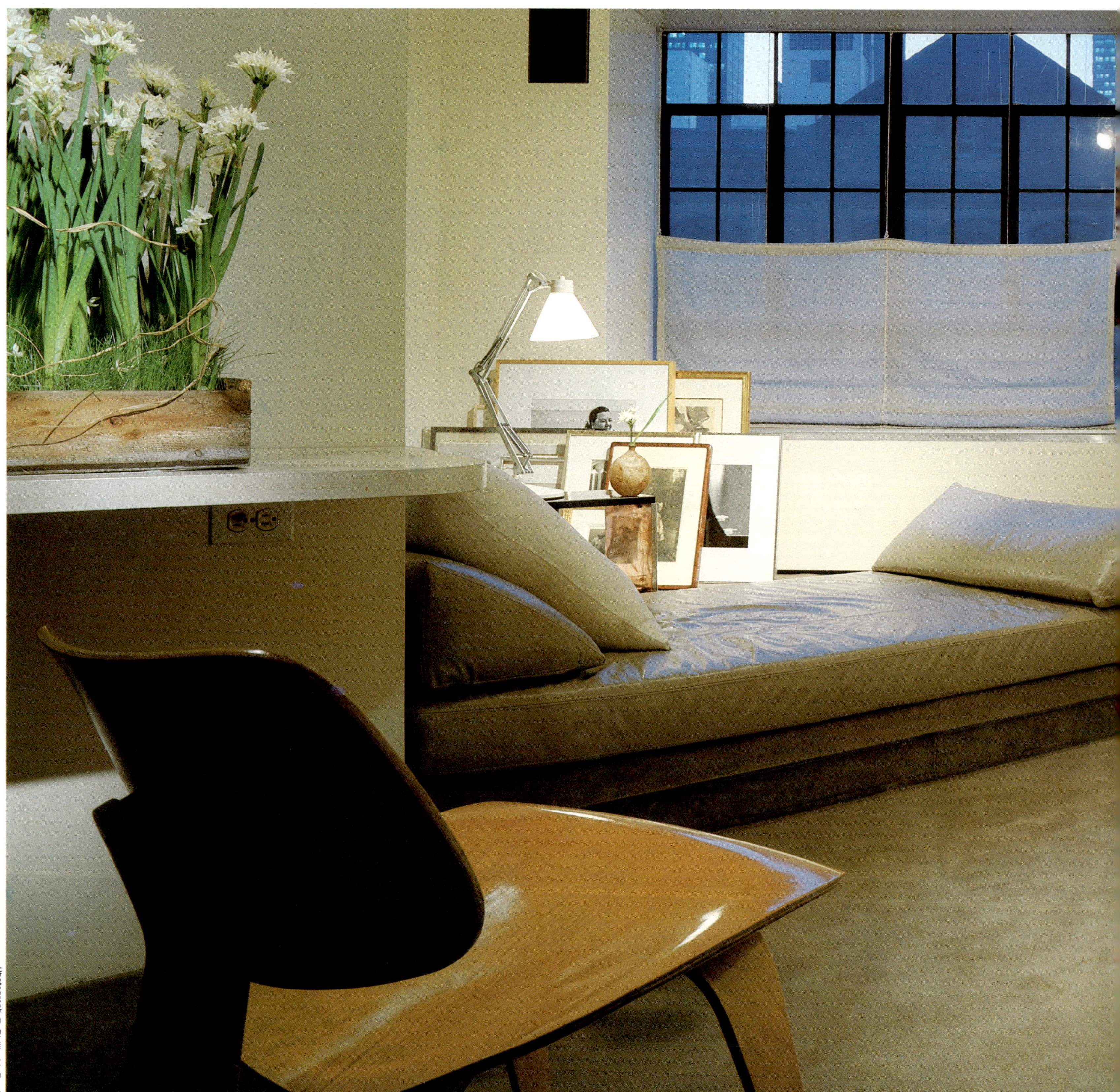

—Photograph © Phillip H. Ennis

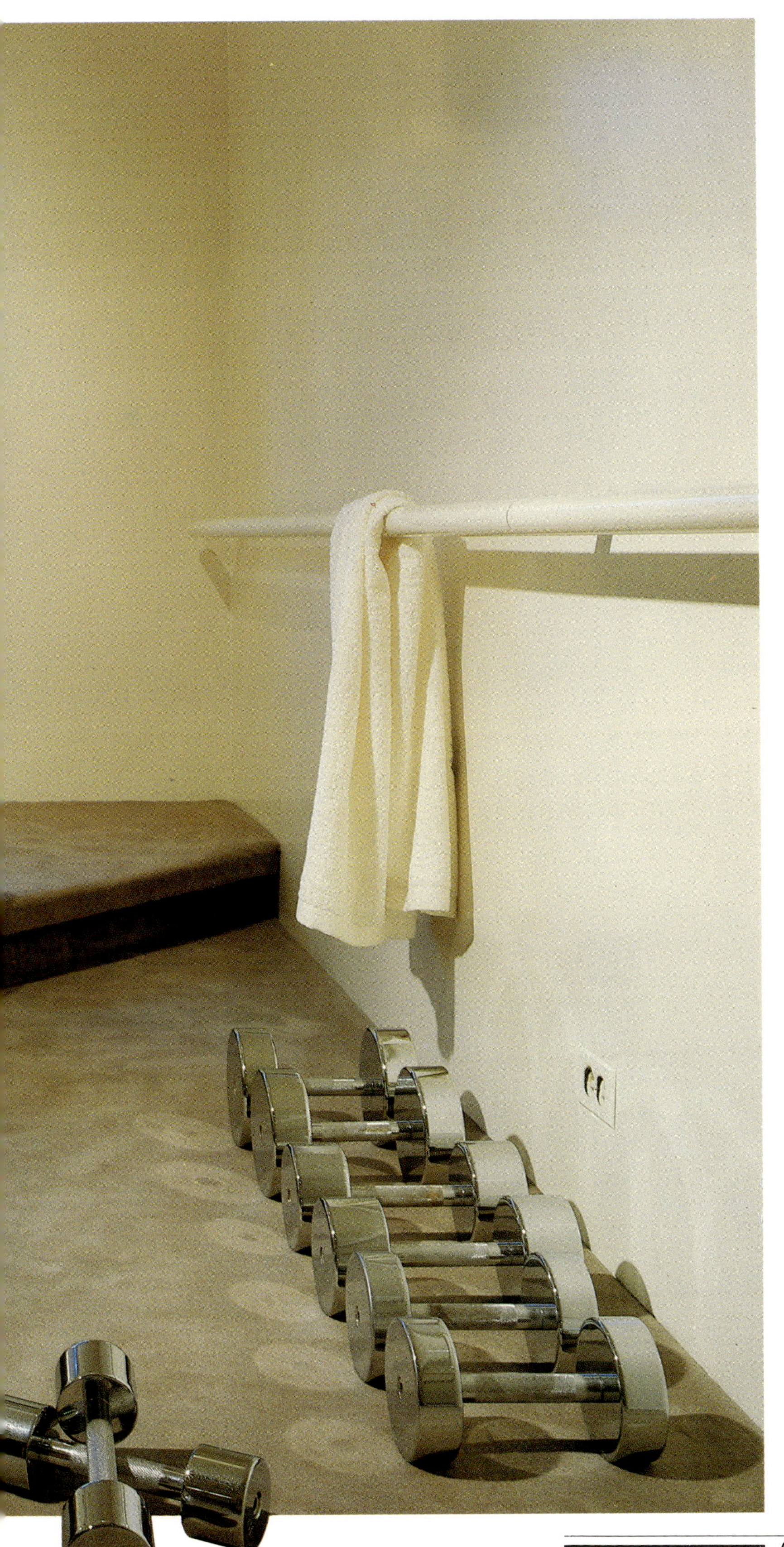

A custom-designed leather cushion and pillows define the post-exercise area of this sleek exercise studio. A Charles Eames moulded plywood chair (c. 1945) strikes a note of mid-century modernism; flushmounted audio speakers flank the mullioned window.

EDITED FOR STYLE

The interiors of Bob Patino and Vincent Wolf resonate with a style and quality seldom encountered in the contemporary idiom; colours, materials, and textures collectively illustrate the fusion of elegance and simplicity. Apparent simplicity can, however, often deceive. Behind this serene facade lies a complex process of selection, elimination, and attention to detail. This type of solution leaves no room for error.

Approaching the space with an architect's concern for structure and spatial relationships, co-designers Patino and Wolf reoriented the room's visual axis with a raised diagonal platform. Replete with leather-covered cushion and pillows, the newly defined corner is perfect for post-exercise relaxation or reading. Plush carpeting counterpoints the slick, reflective walls finished with twenty-seven coats of automobile lacquer. A wall-mounted dancers' barre and a set of chrome-plated dumbbells make up the equipment profile. The overflow of a burgeoning art collection is casually stored in the corner—a confident touch which mitigates the room's otherwise serious nature.

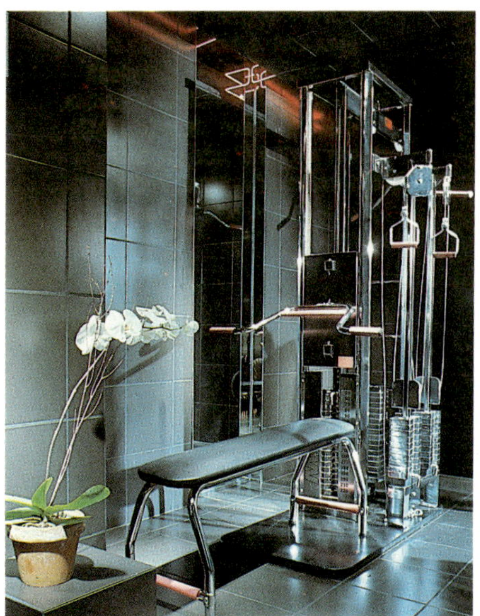

The far wall behind the exercise area contains a flushmounted audio system. Small edge lights enhance subtle architectural details such as the floating shower platform. ▷

A tile-clad column structurally defines the exercise and dressing areas of this spa/bathroom. The glass-enclosed walk-in closet beside the sink features an electronically controlled, recirculating clothes rack. The multistation gym is from Marcy. ◁

EXERCISE AND ENTERTAINMENT

Architectural integrity and intrinsic luxury go hand in hand in this bathroom designed by Eric Bernard. Designed for exercise and entertainment, the space combines bath, spa, dressing room, gym, and media room. Bernard successfully manages functional and aesthetic compatibility with a disciplined gallerylike plan and graphic surface treatment.

A study in planar geometry, the space is organized along its longitudinal axis—a clear central path with amenities arranged along the room's perimeter. The shower, whirlpool, and electronic chaise are on one side, while the multistation gym and dressing table are opposite. The far back wall contains a flushmounted audio system, while the wall beside the sink features a glass-enclosed walk-in closet. Italian ceramic tiles in a matte black finish reiterate the room's disciplined geometry.

A tile-clad column structurally defines the workout zone and dressing area. A television niche over the "floating" sink counter permits convenient viewing, and the nearby control panel interfaces with the lighting, audio, and video systems. Dakota Jackson's hydraulic stool provides just the right touch of industrial chic.

On the opposite side, the glass-enclosed shower and whirlpool tub is adjoined by an electronically controlled chaise for postexercise relaxation. Various lighting modes can illuminate a spectrum of moods from surface-mounted track lights, recessed floods, and even candlelight.

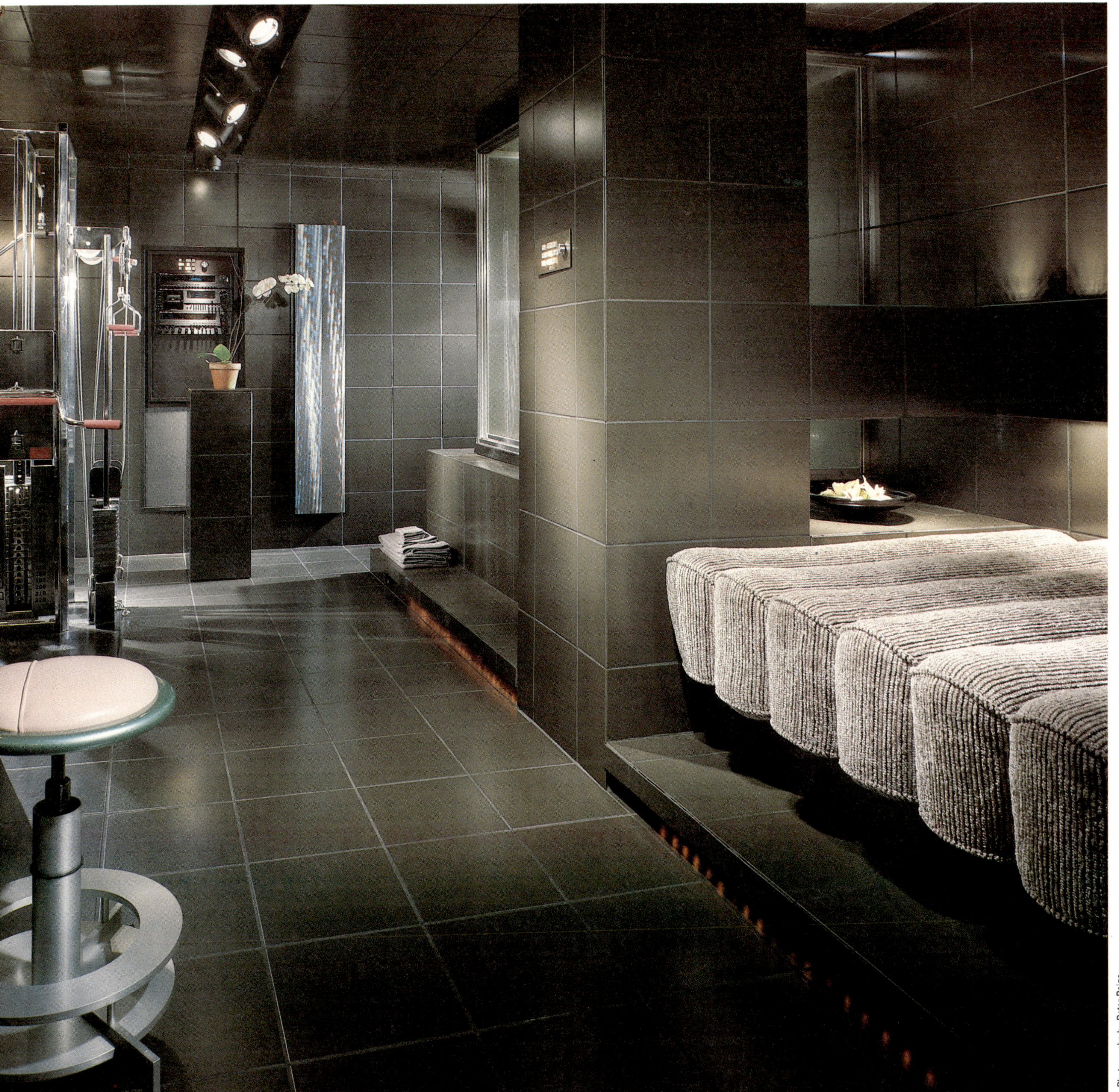

—Photographs by Peter Paige

Flanked by red metal lockers, a black laminate entertainment unit is reflected in the mirrored wall panels. The lockers provide practical storage space for friends' clothes, while the flushmounted television and audio system can either set the pace or provide diversion.

HOME-GROWN LOCKER ROOM

A multifunctional space is intended to fulfill a variety of purposes with equal assurance; ideally, no one activity should visually dominate the room's functional identity. Designed by Samuel Botero Associates, this room successfully meets this criteria by serving as a home gym, entertainment center, and guest quarters: One doesn't disrupt the other.

Located in a postwar high-rise, Botero used deepened window wells and an elevated bed platform to enhance the feeling of structural solidity and add architectural interest. A very original media/storage cabinet is undeniably the room's focal point: Fabricated in black laminate, the unit is flanked by two sets of lacquered metal lockers. Recalling the locker room of a high school or health club, the solution is as witty as it is practical. Guests who work out with the resident can conveniently store their belongings in the lockers. They'll also be able to enjoy the luxury of an audio/video system.

Since the client is committed to a program of weight training, the equipment profile includes a set of chrome-plated dumbbells and stainless caddy, an extended curl bar with chromed weight plates, and a supine bench.

The restrained color palette is sparked with bold colorful pillows on the bed; with pure decorative élan, Botero covered the supine bench to match the pillows. An industrial-grade carpeting was chosen for its clean good looks and durability.

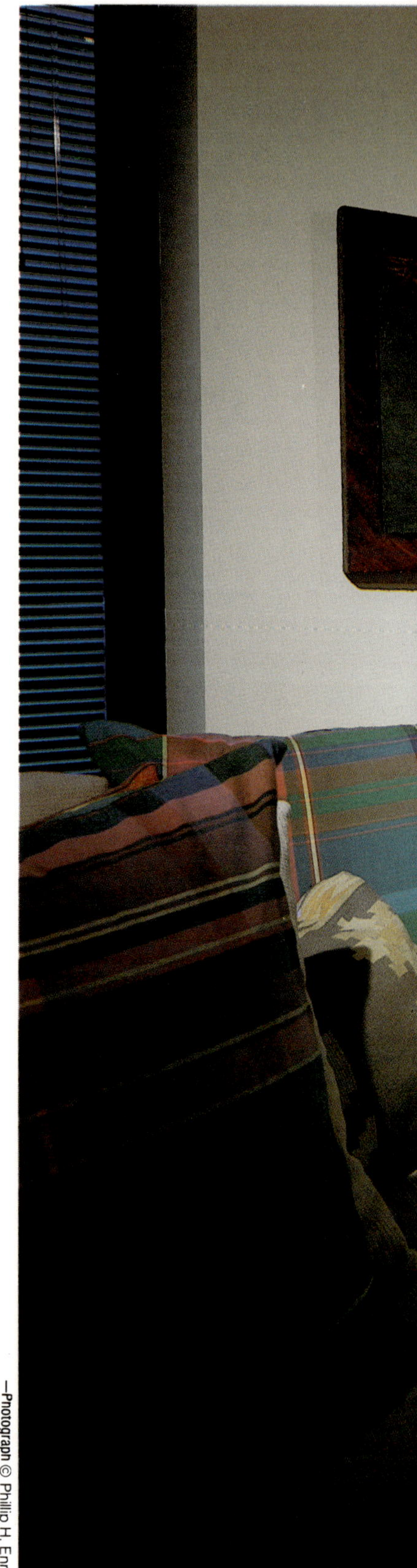

—Photograph © Phillip H. Ennis

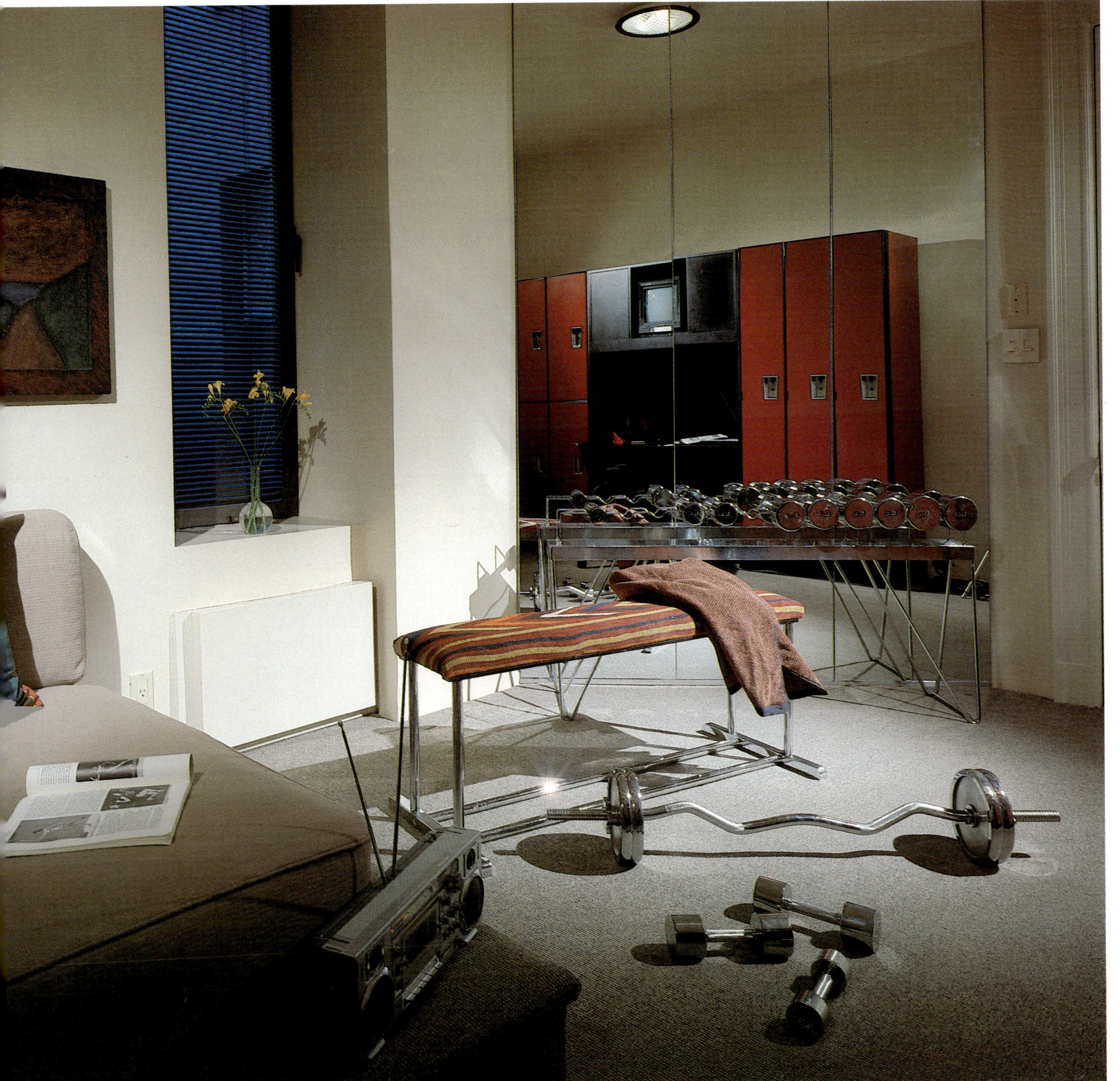

A custom-designed étagère features a system of milled cradles that respond perfectly to the dumbbells' graduated sizes. An oak border around the perimeter of the room defines the workout zone and maintains its residential character. ▷

Mirror panels (inset) behind the oak dancer's barre feature an applied cornice fitted with an uplight. The multistation gym, exercise mat, and dancer's barre share space with a stationary bicycle and mounted punching bag.

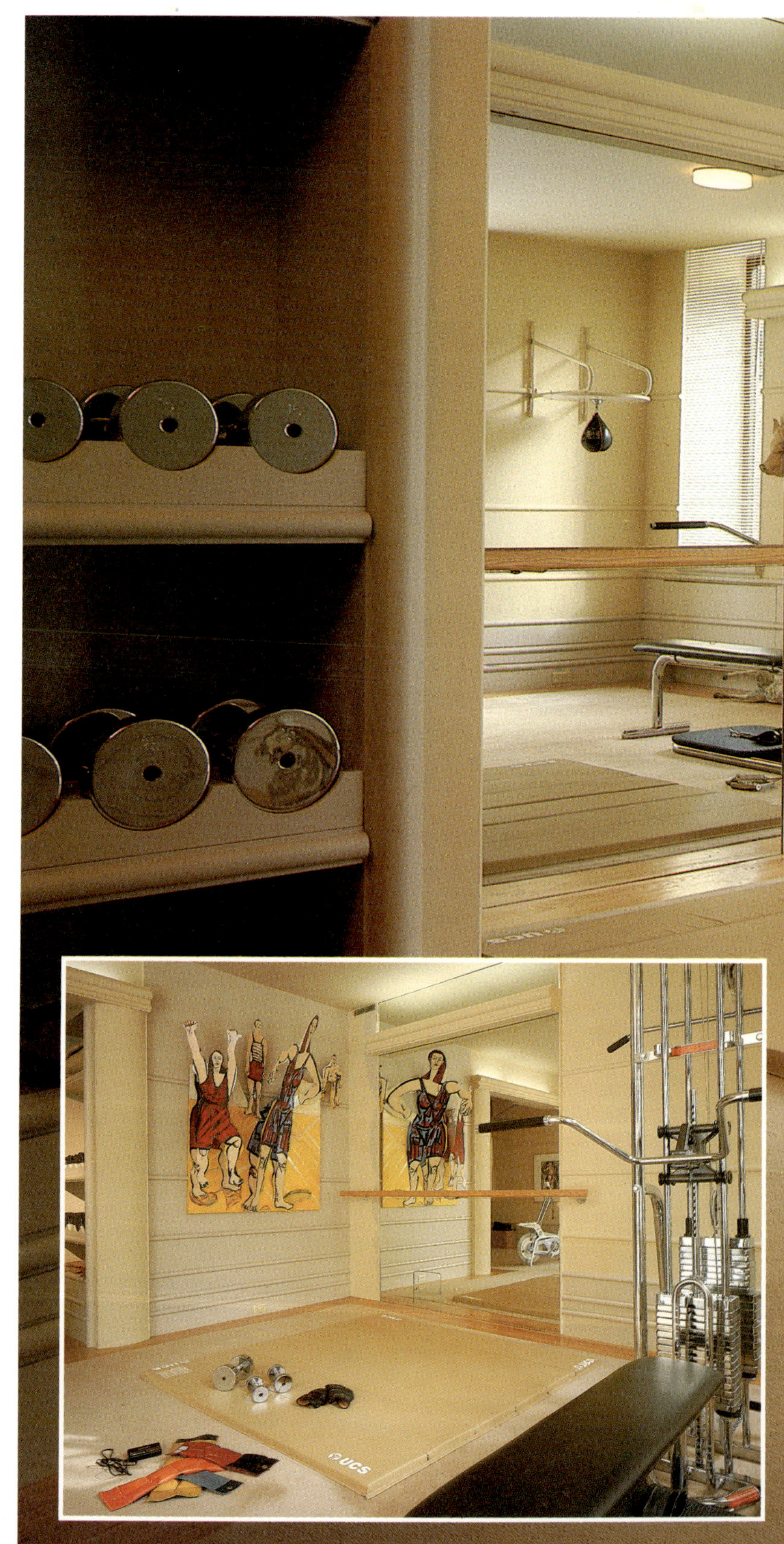

MODULOR THEORY

A surface treatment of applied moldings, cornices, and lintels reflects architect Michael Mostoller's personal interpretation of classical ornamentation and proportion. With sensitive detailing and coloration, Mostoller manages the considerable task of maintaining the room's residential character without eclipsing the function for which it was planned.

In addition to personal expression, the architect skillfully uses ornamentation to create architectural illusion. Based on Le Corbusier's *Modulor 2* treatise, panel molding was applied in platonic mathematical ratios in which increments are calculated by simply adding the one in front. A sample progression would follow as 1 2 3 5 8 13... ad infinitum.

The graduated moldings are used to almost encourage the resident up to greater heights both physically and metaphorically. For practicality, Mostoller employs such architectural devices to force the illusion of symmetry within an essentially asymmetrical space. The dropped cornices, centered over the mirror and between the windows, for example, significantly enhance the room's grandeur and symmetry.

Planned for a devoted enthusiast, the room is light, spacious, and well-equipped. Exercise amenities include a chrome-plated multistation gym, a stationary bicycle, an exercise mat, and a dancer's barre. There is also a mounted punching bag and large sauna.

A custom-designed étagère by the entrance features a unique system of milled cradles perfectly corresponding to the various sized dumbbells they contain. For definition, Mostoller outlined the carpeted workout zone with an oak border—adding surface interest and once again reiterating the room's residential character.

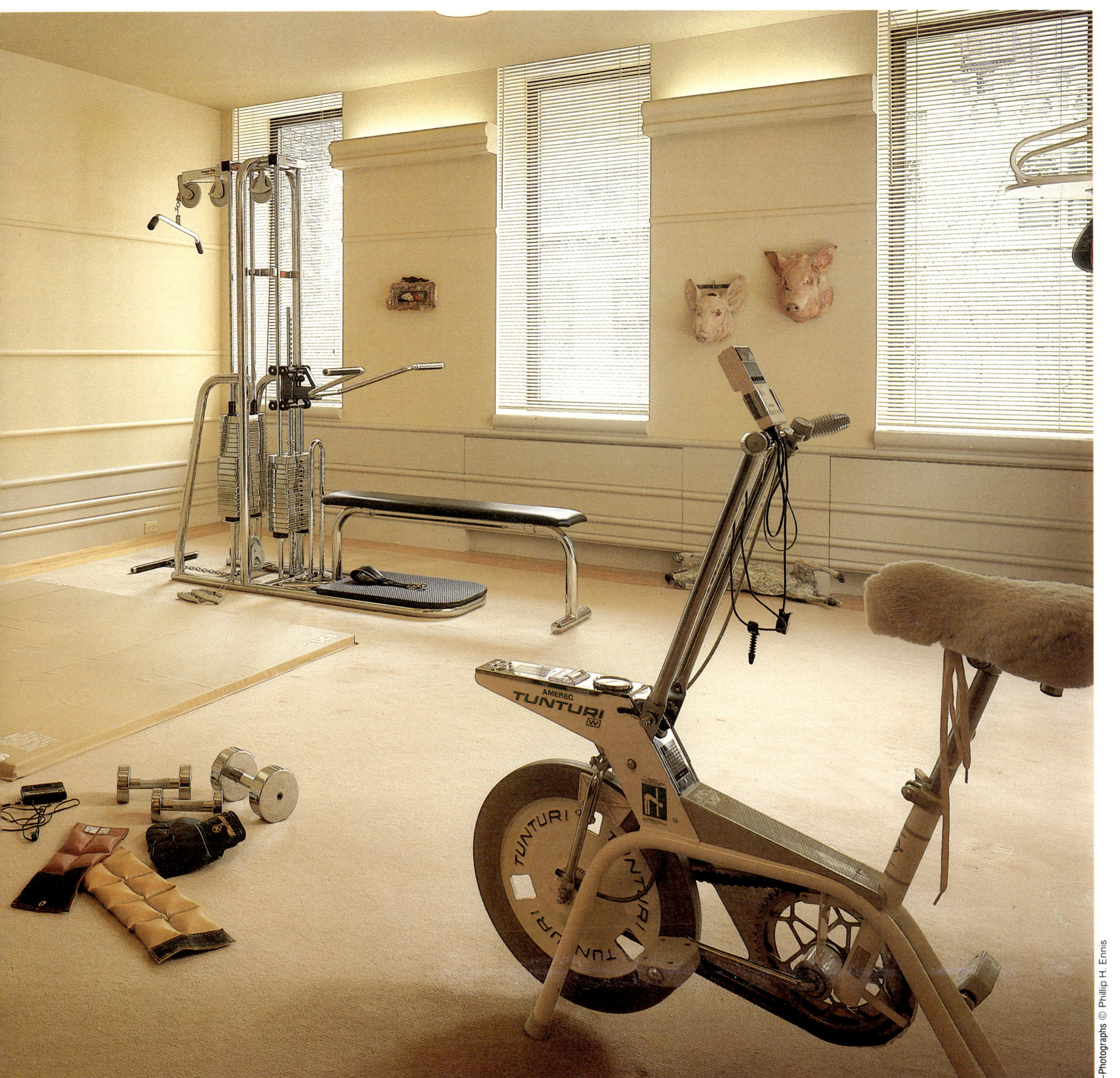

—Photographs © Phillip H. Ennis

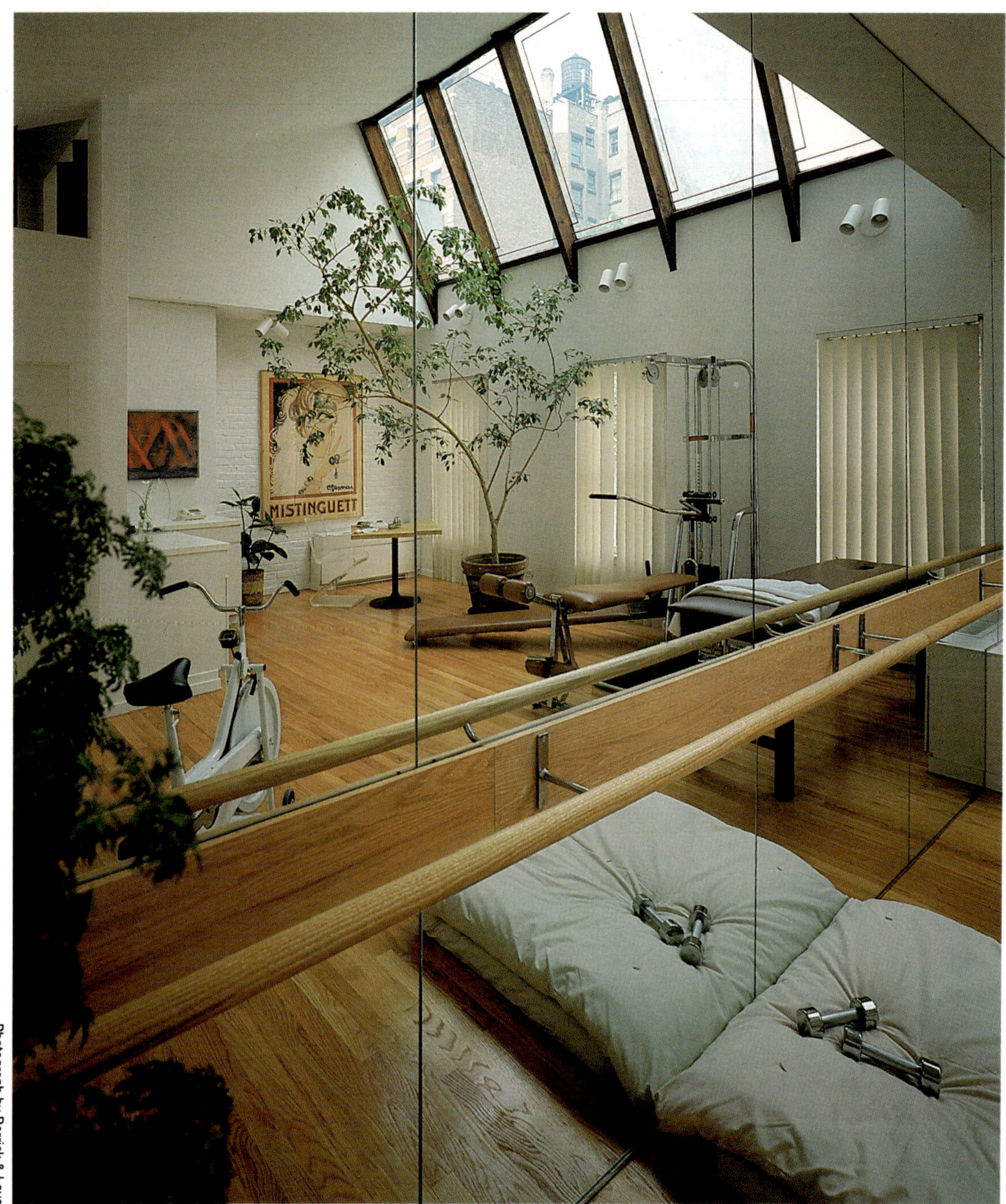

—Photograph by Derrick & Love

PENT-HOUSE GYM

An oak dancers' barre spans the mirror-clad wall of this penthouse gymnasium. A convenient snack-bar kitchen is tucked away in a corner, while a large-angled skylight amplifies the space with a rooftop view.

A soaring, light-filled space, this penthouse gymnasium sits unexpectedly atop a New York City high-rise. Originally conceived as a dancer's studio, its white walls and bare floors provided a serene, distraction-free environment for its resident dancer. The space was therefore equipped only with a dancers' barre, exercise mat, and mirrored wall.

Designer Engle Yokley softened the room's austerity with a cozy snack-bar kitchen, wood-trimmed skylight, and nineteenth-century French cabaret poster. As her clients' interests grew to include a complete fitness programme, additional equipment was purchased. With an eye for both aerobic and anaerobic exercises, the equipment profile grew to include a stationary bicycle, slant board, multi-station gym, massage table, and chrome-plated dumbbell set.

ARCHITECTURAL GRID LOCK

David Eugene Bell, ASID and Donald Cotter of Design Multiples designed this bath with an eye toward fitness and relaxation. Cobalt-blue Italian ceramic tiles with white grouting effectively reiterate the room's geometry with the added bonus of durability and easy maintenance.

Two adjoining elevations define functional areas within the space. A less-than-full-height partition encloses the whirlpool bath in its own cozy niche two steps above the built-in chaise. Fitted with a towel-clad cushion, the chaise doubles as an exercise aid and comfortable relaxing spot. The horizontal sink counter is fronted by plain mirror panels that open to reveal considerable storage space, while the small open étagère displays those more aesthetically compatible necessities.

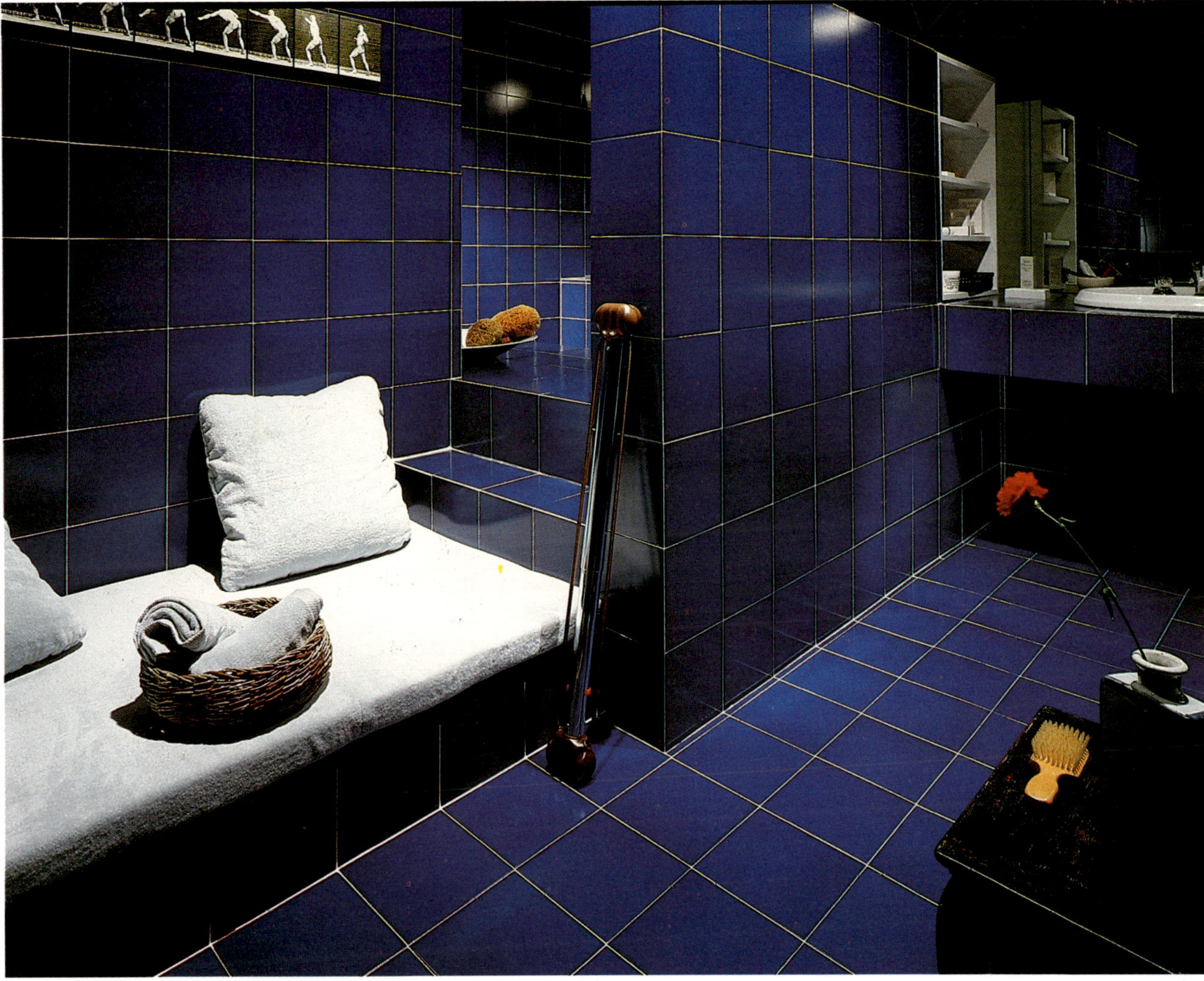

—Photograph by Siesel Co.

The white-cushioned built-in chaise with an isometric compression bar, comfortably assists workouts while doubling as a private corner for reading and relaxing. Stairs lead to an elevated whirlpool bath concealed by the tiled partition.

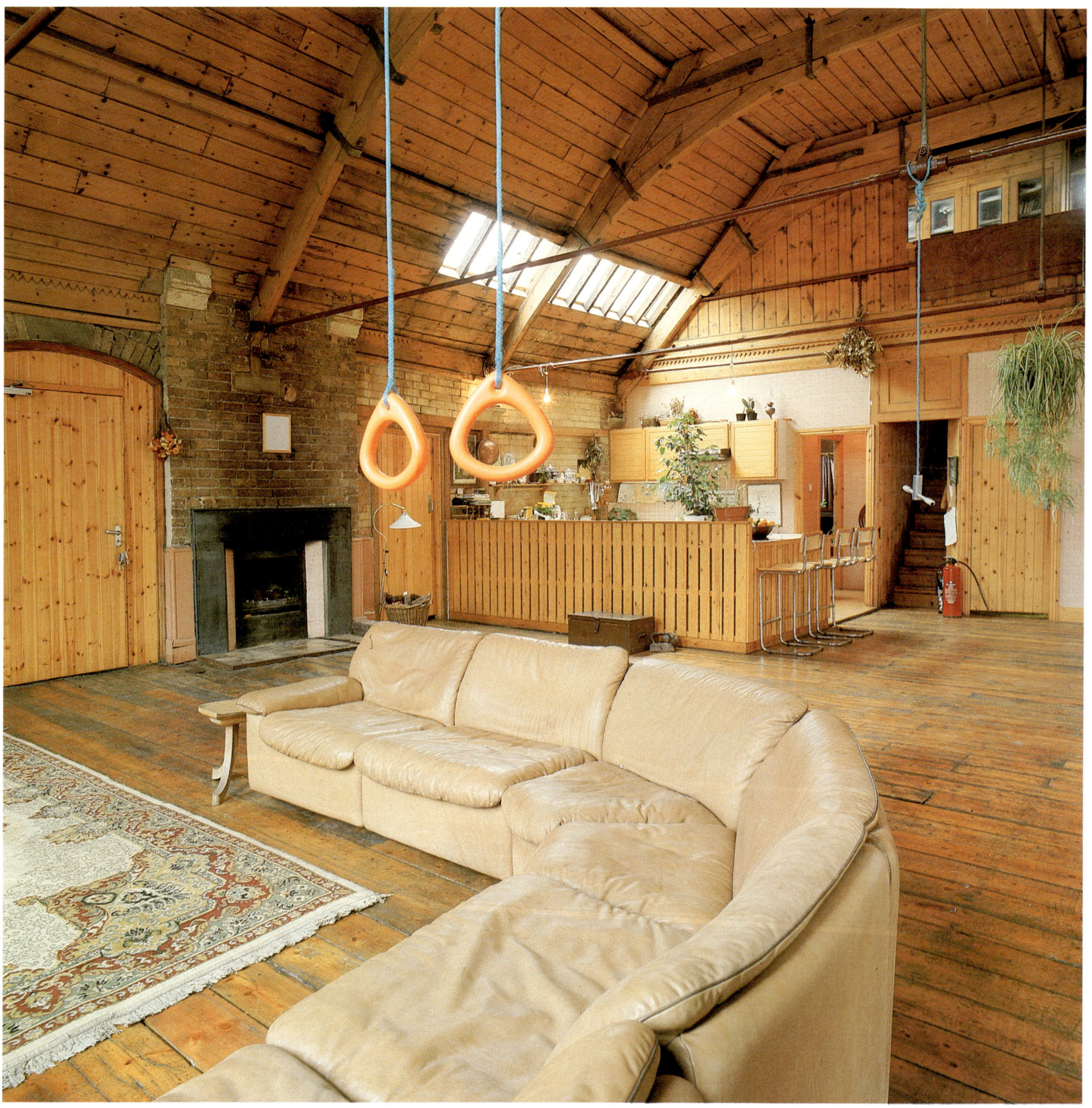

—Photographs © Morley Von Sternberg

◁ **Exercise rings and trapeze bars assume a more sociable character in this domestic setting when the residents' guests playfully challenge their strength and endurance. The open-plan kitchen respects the integrity and materials of the original space.**

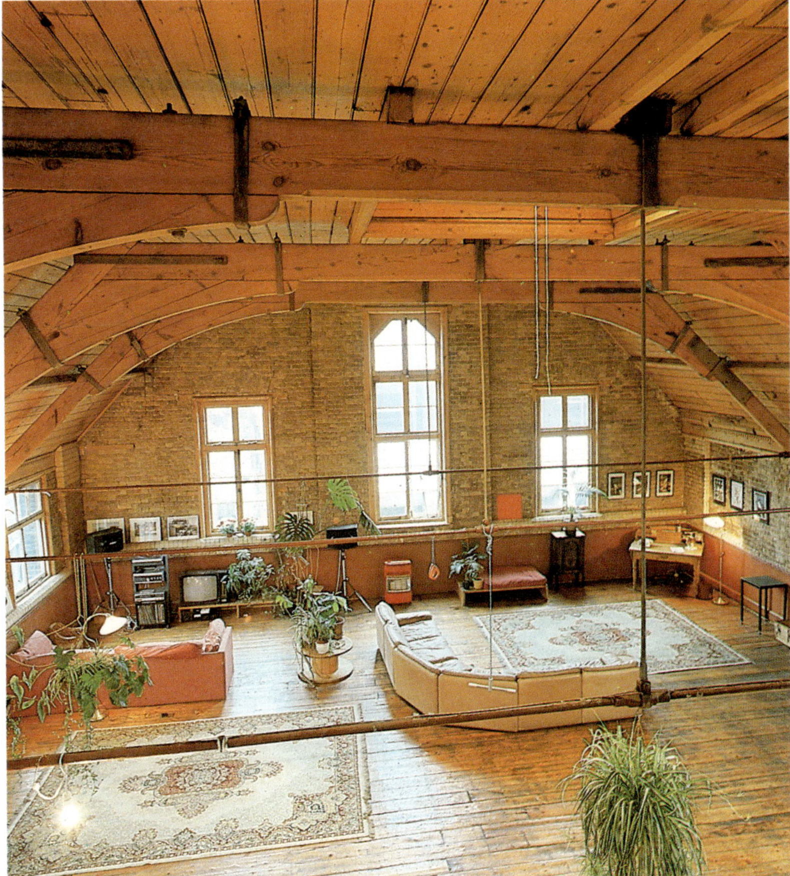

◁ **The timber-vaulted room of this London mews house adds a note of structural grandeur. Seating is arranged in two distinct functional groups—a curved modular unit for conversation and a pink-covered sofa for convenient television viewing.**

MASTERFUL MEWS

The strictures normally associated with one-room living are noticably absent in this huge timber-vaulted space. This once-abandoned mews in a now-fashionable London side street has been reincarnated with a plan of careful restoration and decoration.

The clients, who acted as their own designers and artisans, have managed the rudiments of medieval house planning with a great hall for the general use of the entire household, supplemented with private apartments at each end. Since the clients are devoted to a gymnastics programme, the space is equipped only with exercise rings, a climbing rope, and a trapeze T-bar, all suspended from the rafters. Mats are generally used for safety and comfort when dismounting.

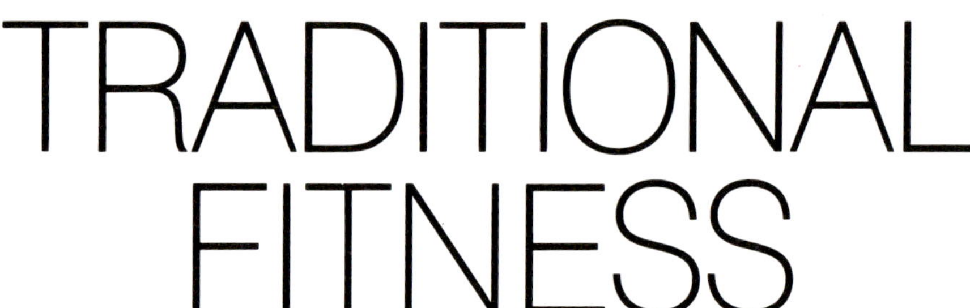

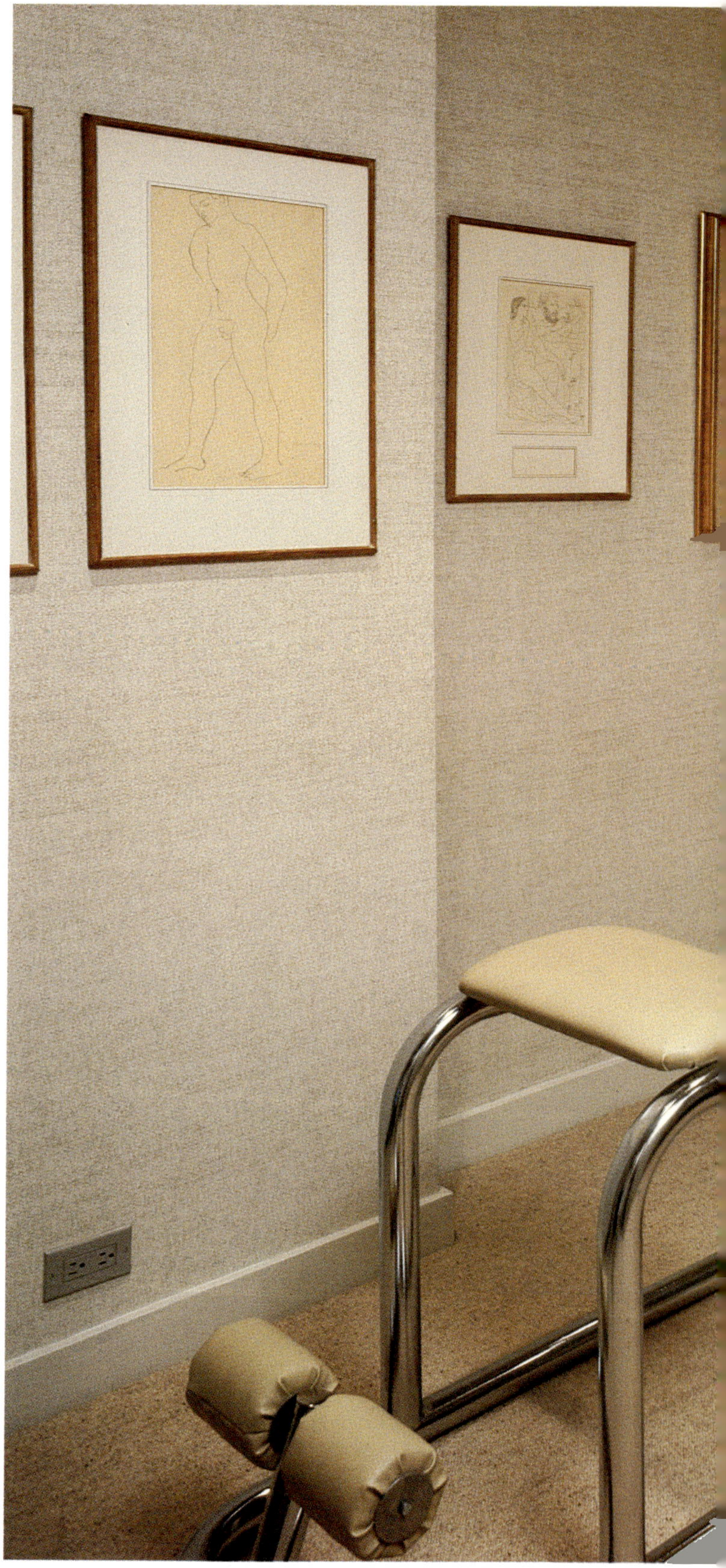

TRADITIONAL FITNESS

Soft grey walls and gilt-framed Picasso etchings set a tone of unexpected elegance in this home gym designed by Richard Debnam Lawrence for songwriter/producer Jack Lawrence. The space is equipped with a wall-mounted, multi-use gym; stationary bicycle; abdominal stool with ankle rollers; and isometric compression bar. Contact surfaces have all been custom-upholstered in soft beige glove leather. The carpeted floor is backed with an extra-thick foam pad, eliminating the need for exercise mats.

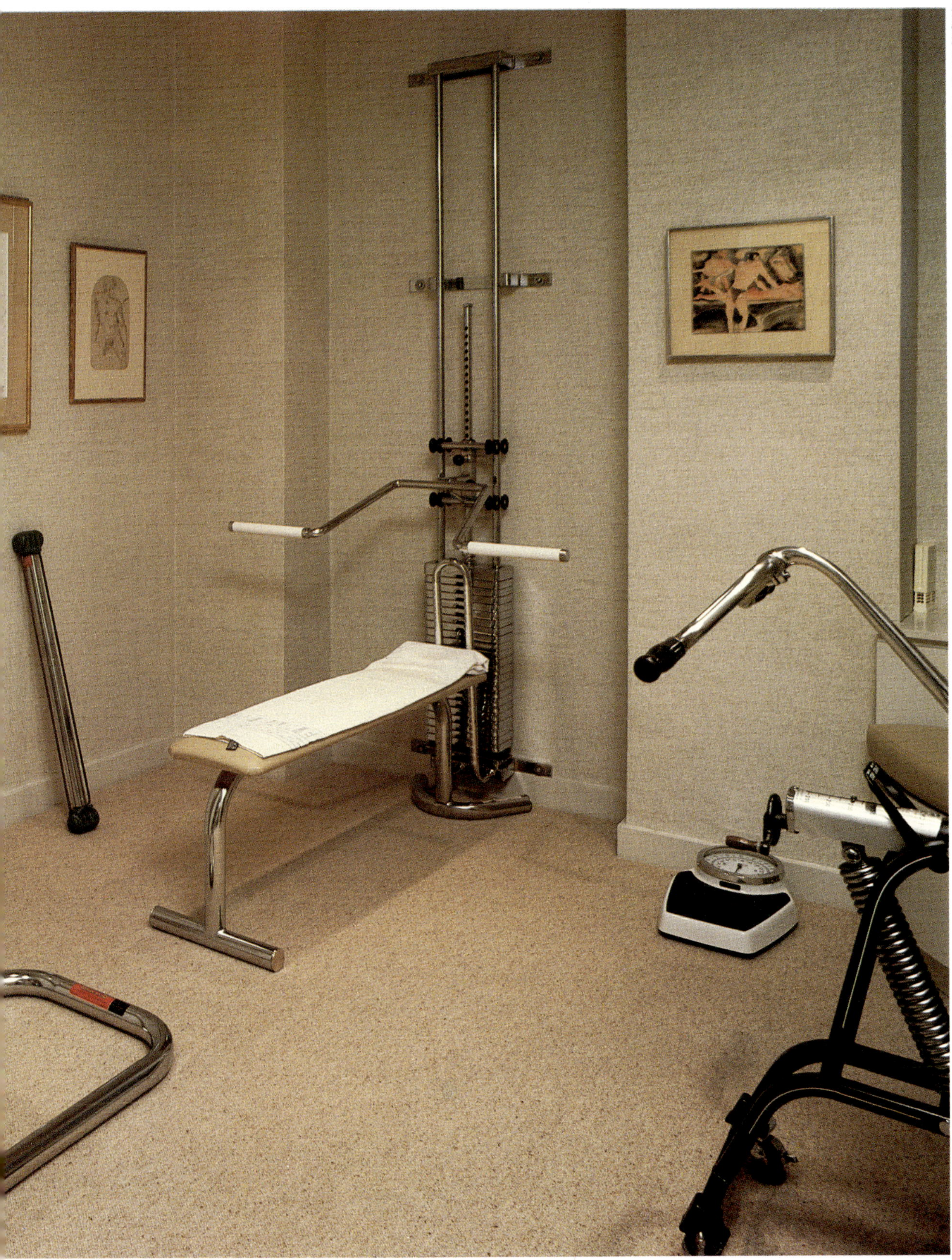

—Photograph by Norman McGrath

Designer Lawrence created this gym with an eye to visual compatibility with the rest of his client's maisonette—hence the elegant colour scheme and gilt-framed etchings. The nickel-plated equipment—with custom-covered contact surfaces—has been arranged to suit the client's preferred routine.

The gym in fashion designer Adri's loft shares space with the sleeping and dressing area. A wall of floor-to-ceiling mirror panels backs the dancer's barre and camouflages a set of mismatched windows. Exercise rings by AMF, an exercise mat, and cast-iron dumbbells complete the equipment profile. The carpeted platform sports a leather-covered mattress.

A massive white-tiled pool ▷ platform is the architectural mainstay of the loft. Designer Walz angled the square whirlpool to offset its rigid geometry and enhance the view. The platform also conceals plumbing, kitchen storage, and a dressing table.

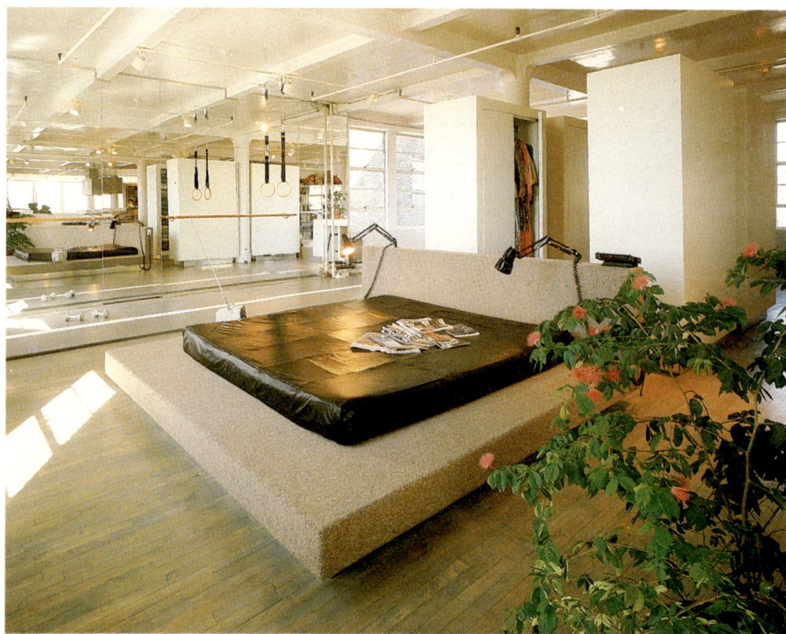

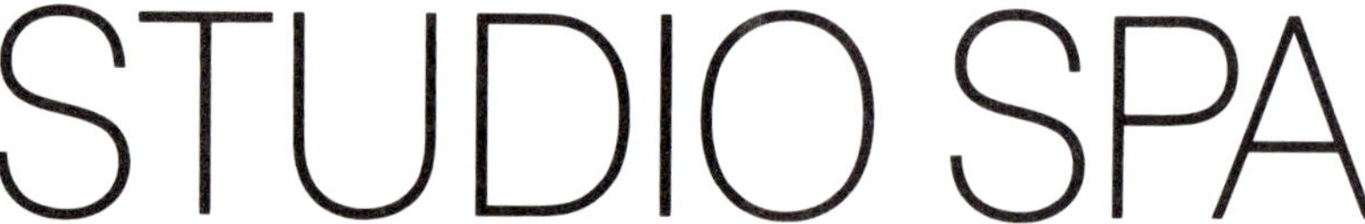

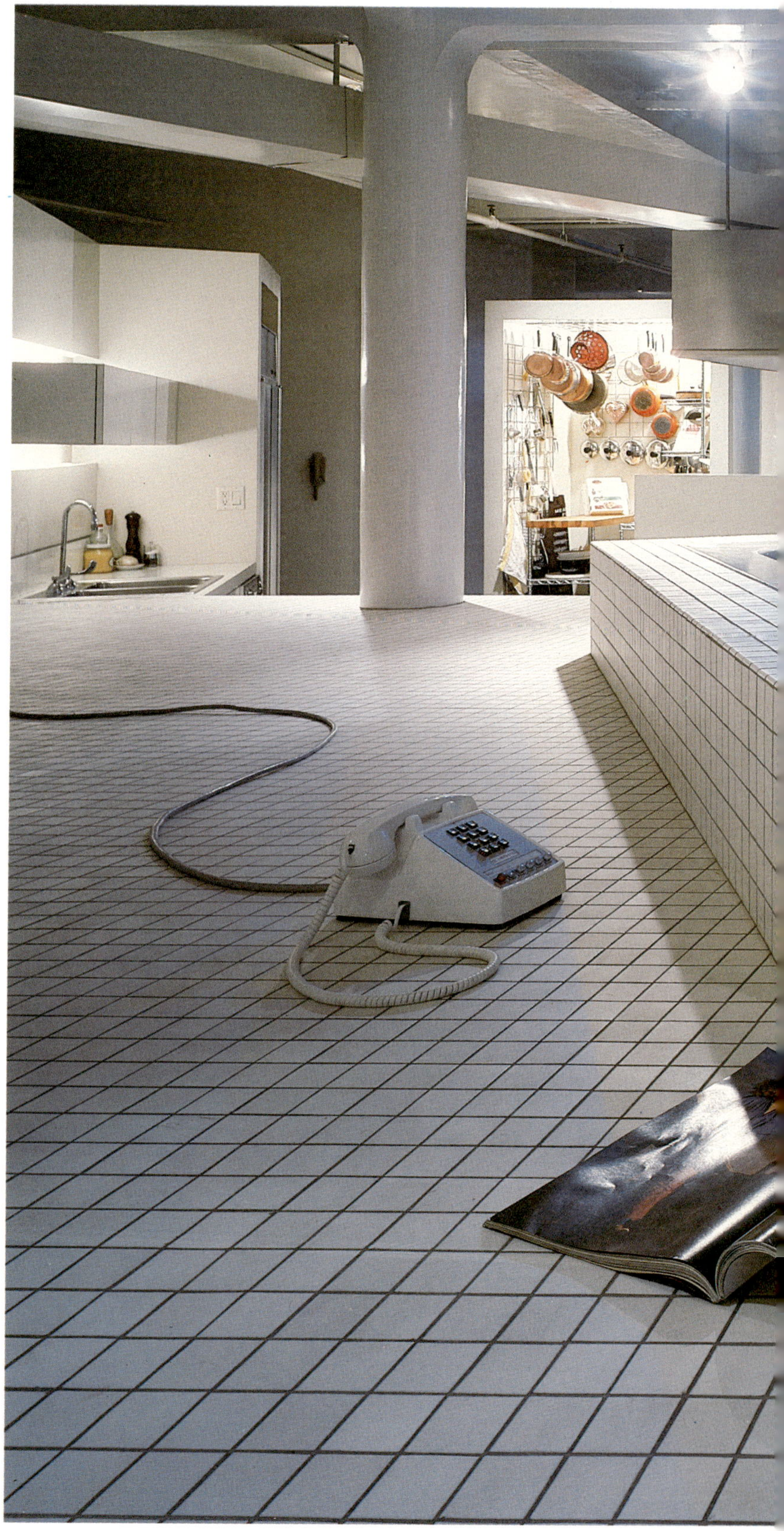

STUDIO SPA

When fashion designer Adri purchased her lower Manhattan loft, her requirements were clear: one huge, open living, dining, and sleeping area complete with gym and swimming pool. Designer Kevin Walz met the challenge with his functional yet stylish approach. To prevent the loft from seeming too large (it is 4,000 square feet), Walz anchored the space with massive architectural elements such as the overscaled pool platform, kitchen island, and several open closets on wheels. While realizing the idea of a gymnasium was easily accomplished, a swimming pool would have required an engineering miracle and phenomenal expense. Both designer and his client settled on an oversized whirlpool large enough to float in, yet small enough to qualify as a tub under the building code.

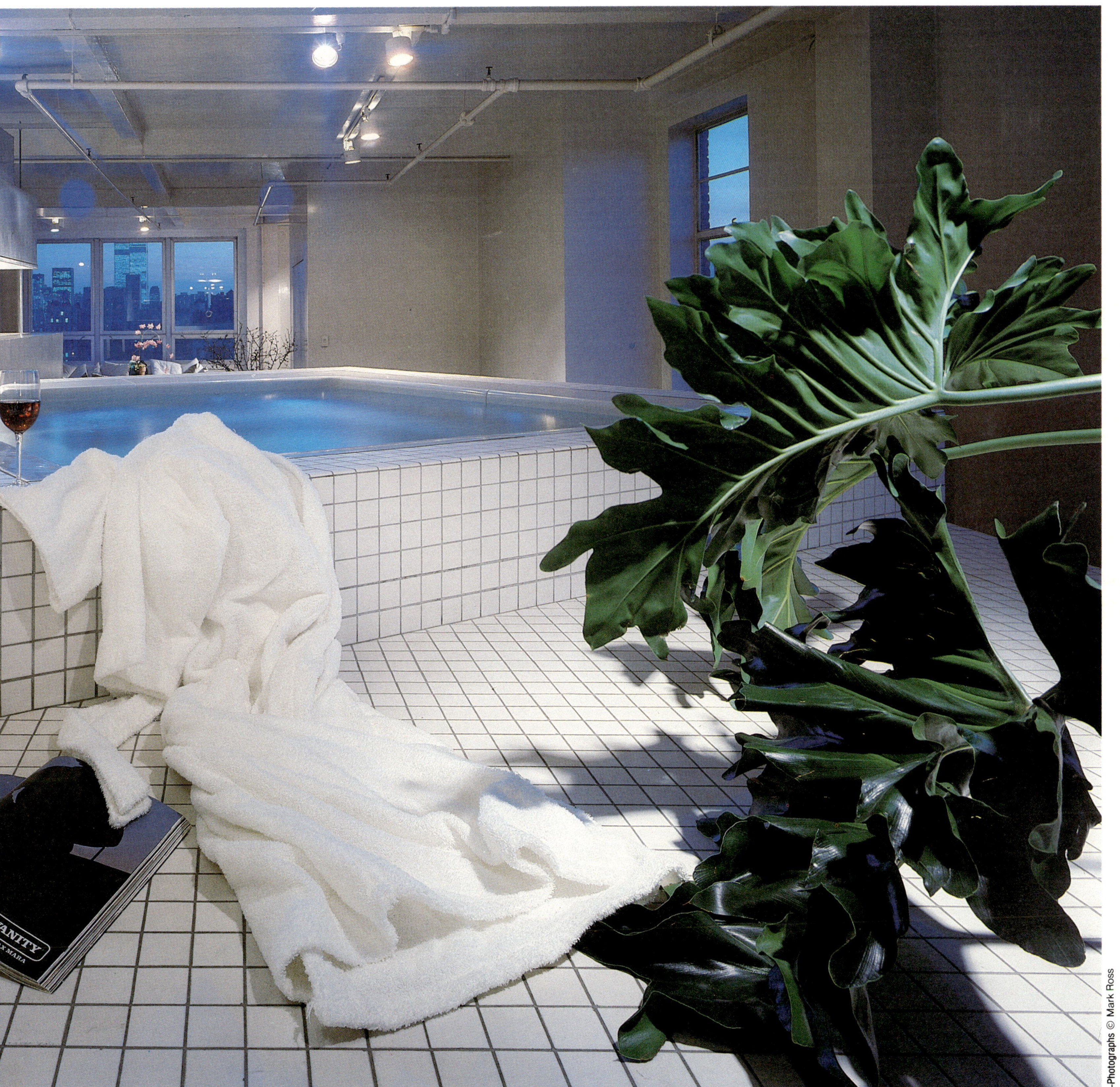

—Photographs © Mark Ross

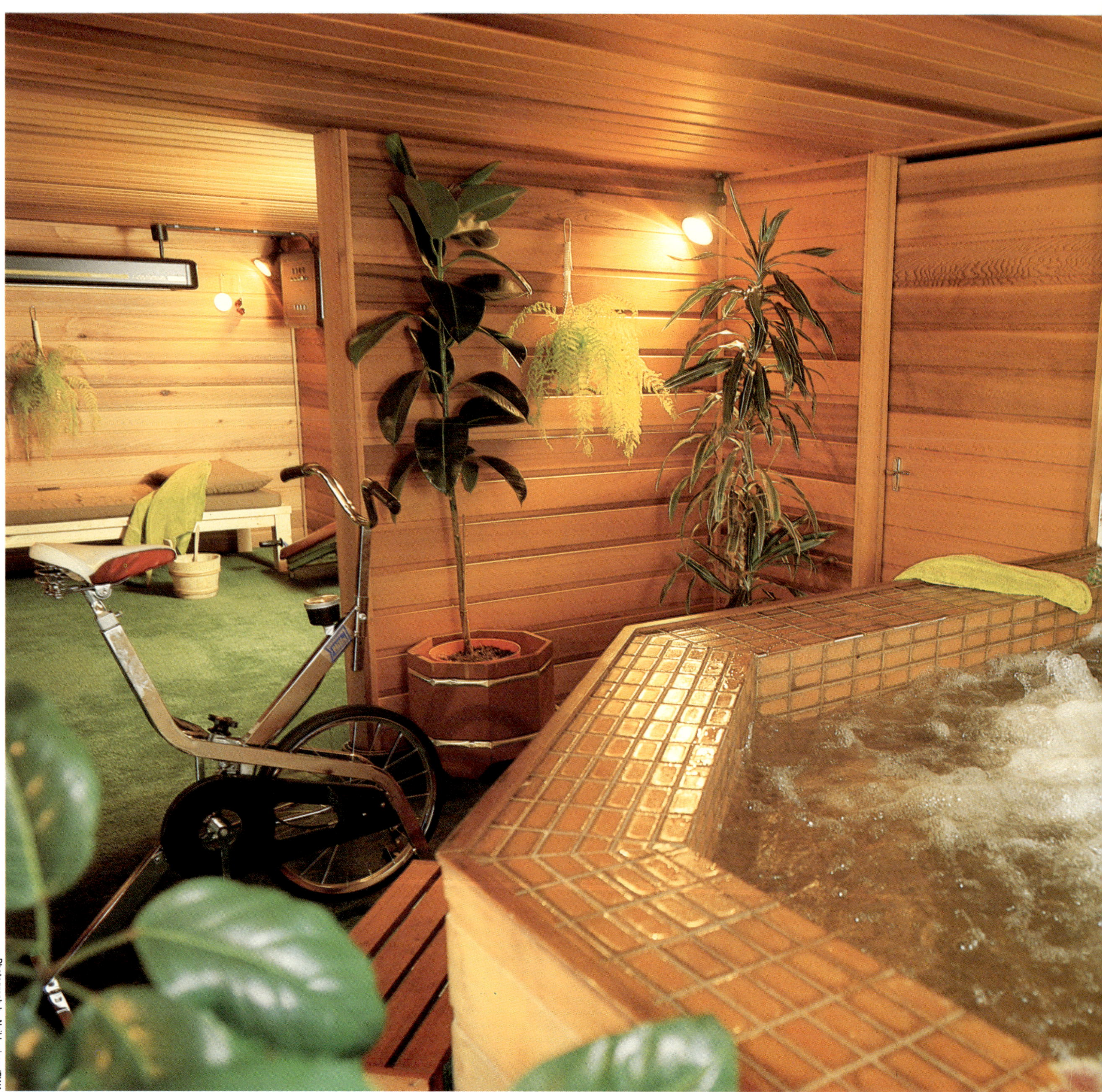

—Photograph by Neil Lorimar/EWA

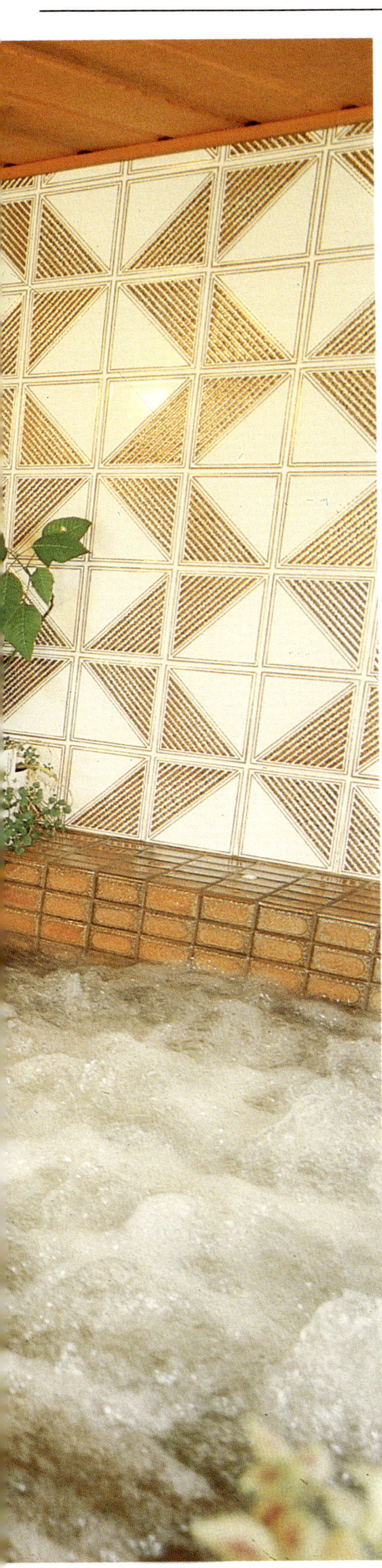

REDWOOD SUITE

A hexagonal tile-covered whirlpool bath is the mainstay of this two-room fitness centre. A separate weight-training and aerobics room contains a low Finnish massage table and a ceiling-mounted ultraviolet tanning lamp.

With its warm colours and redwood planking, this home gymnasium suite borrows design elements from the traditional Finnish bath. A custom-designed hexagonal whirlpool tub takes centre stage in its own anteroom. Covered with narrow Mexican ceramic tiles, the tub is also surrounded by a slatted redwood bench; a stationary bicycle and sauna complete the room's amenities.

Also panelled in redwood, the second room contains all the weight-training equipment. There is also a low, wooden Finnish massage table fitted with a cushion that doubles as a training mat when set on the floor. An ultraviolet tanning lamp is ceiling-mounted above the table. In this room moss-green carpeting was laid over thick foam padding.

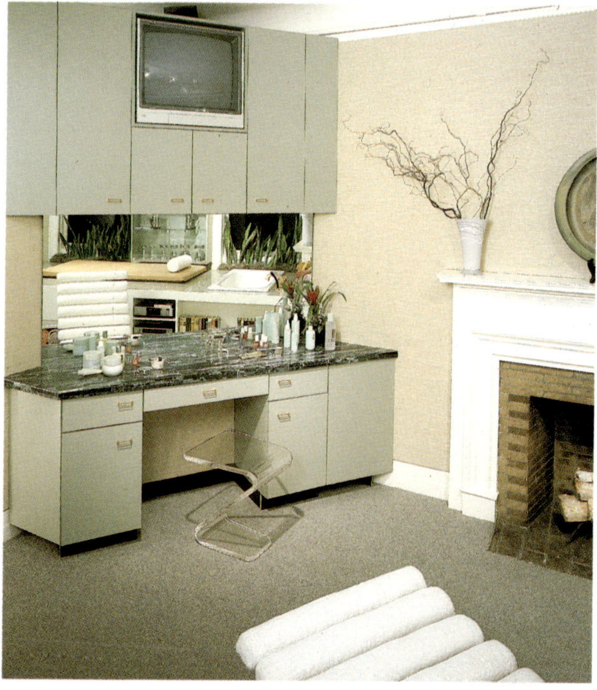

△
A marble-topped dressing table occupies a corner beside the white period chimneypiece. Overhead cabinetry features a 25-inch Sony Profeel monitor, positioned for easy viewing from either the chaise or bath.

COMPATIBLY ZONED

For this sybaritic retreat, designer Rus Calder saw to his clients' fitness as well as entertainment needs. Occupying the space of a former bedroom, it incorporates three functionally compatible zones: one for working out, one for dressing, and one for relaxing.

The fitness zone is defined by an elevated platform along the back wall. A therapeutic whirlpool bath, exercise mat, equipment cabinet, and dancer's barre allow for a varied program of exercise and physical therapy. A tiled surface treatment was selected for its beauty as well as durability.

The carpeted lower level is devoted to less strenuous pursuits. A freestanding dressing table of Calder's own design features a black marble countertop and pair of light fluted columns. The same materials are repeated in the corner dressing table, enlivened by a flushmounted Sony monitor in its overhead canopy. Planned for convenient viewing from either the chaise or the bath, the monitor is equipped with wireless remote control for the ultimate in convenience. Open shelving under the workout platform cleverly stores an audio system, a videocassette recorder, and a small library.

Amenities on the tiled workout platform include a whirlpool bath, exercise mat, and dancer's barre. A matched set of chrome dumbbells, gravity boots, and pulsimeter are visible through the glass doors of the custom-designed storage cabinet. ▷

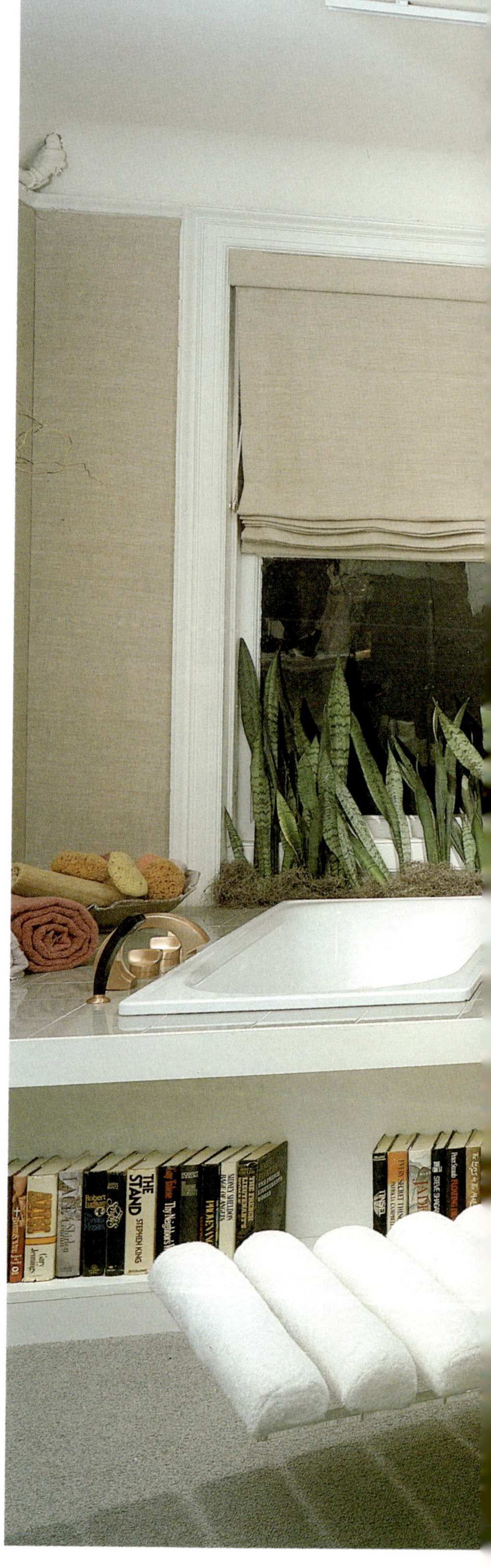

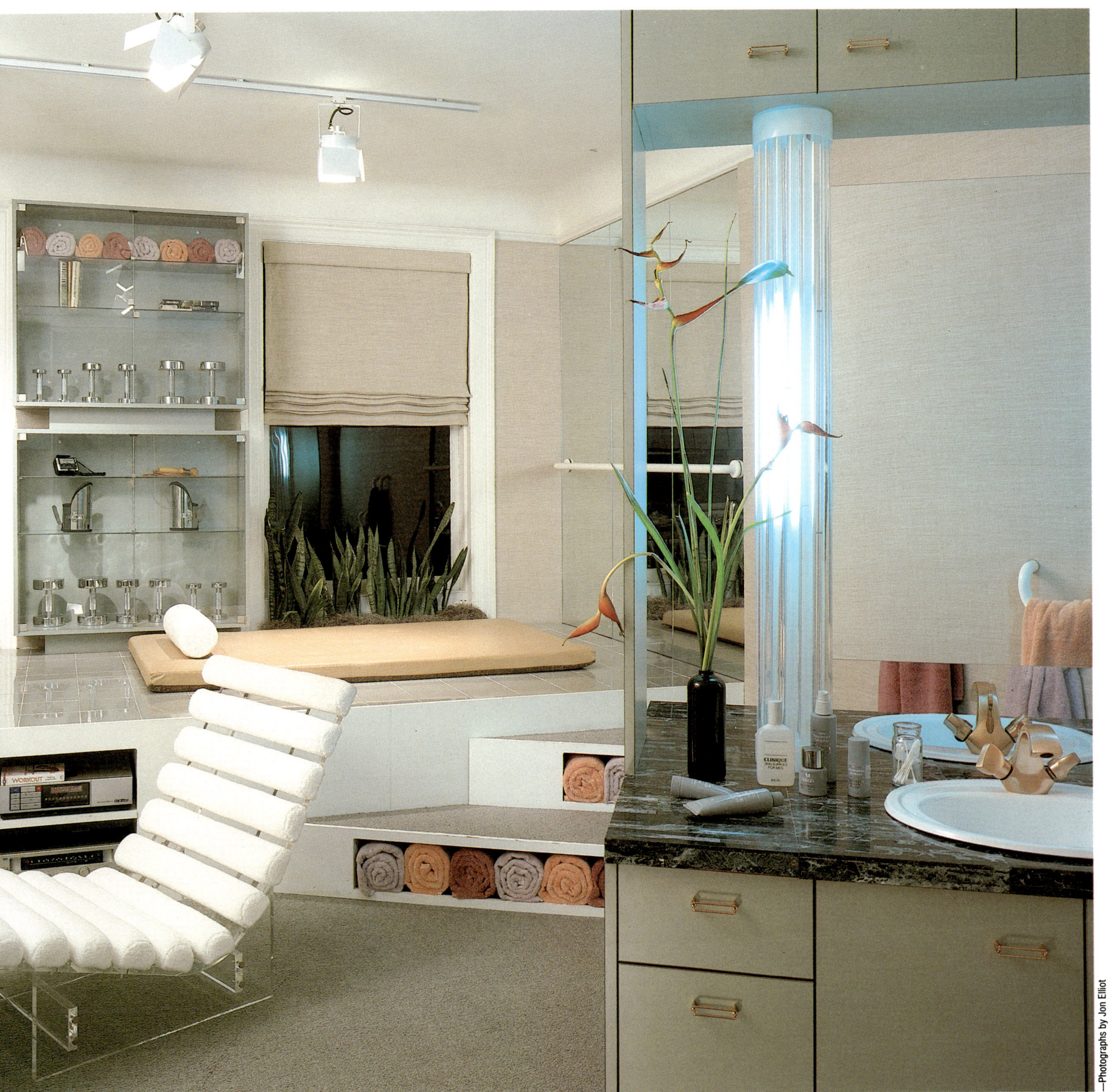

—Photographs by Jon Elliot

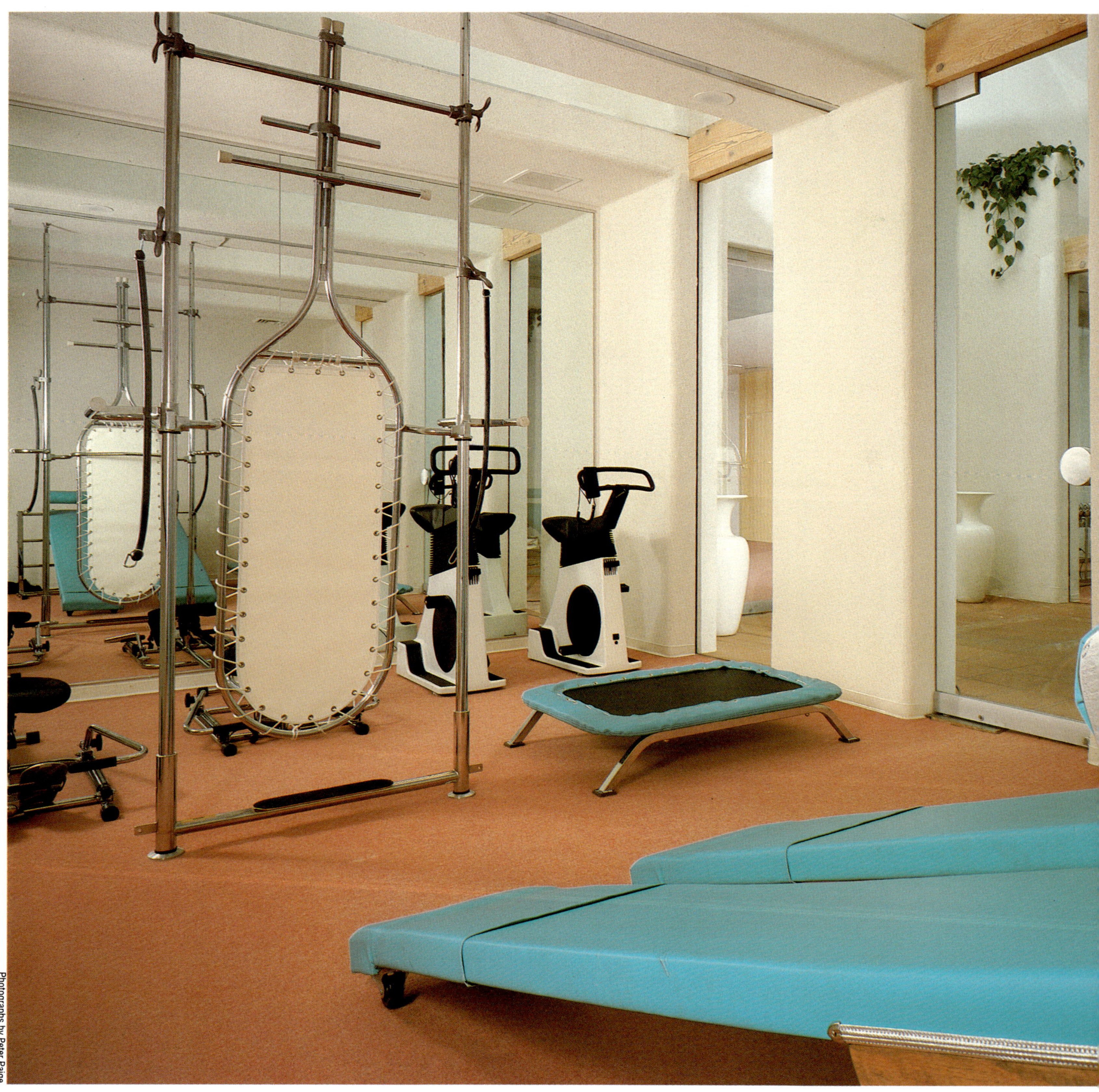

Photographs by Peter Paige

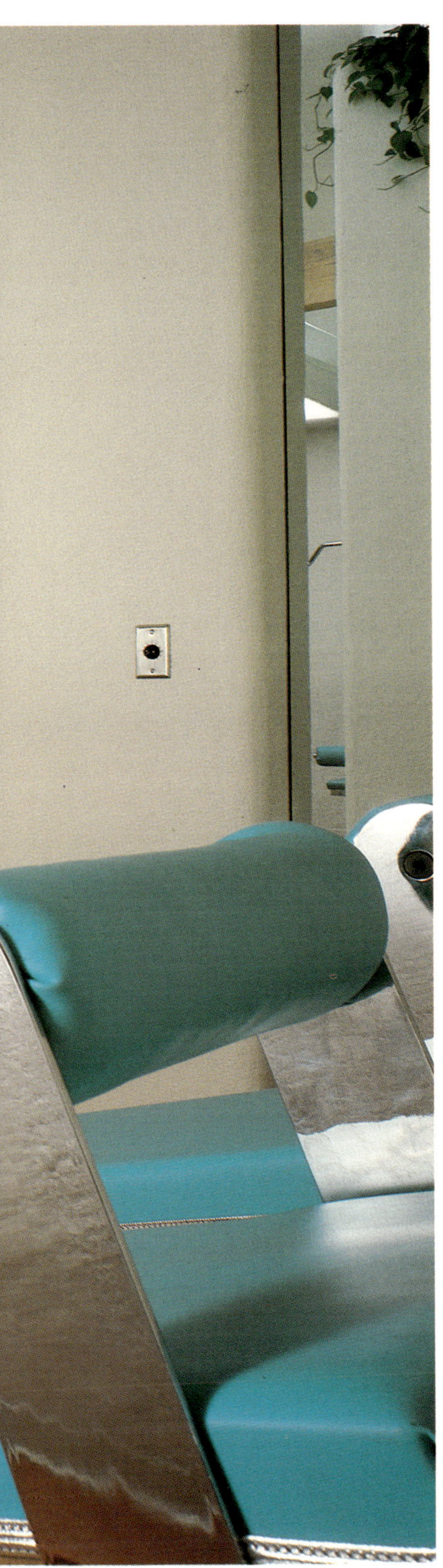

◁ **Exercise equipment is made more vibrant with leather covers in bright turquoise. Recessed mirror panels and long skylights enhance the illusion of intrinsic architectural character.**

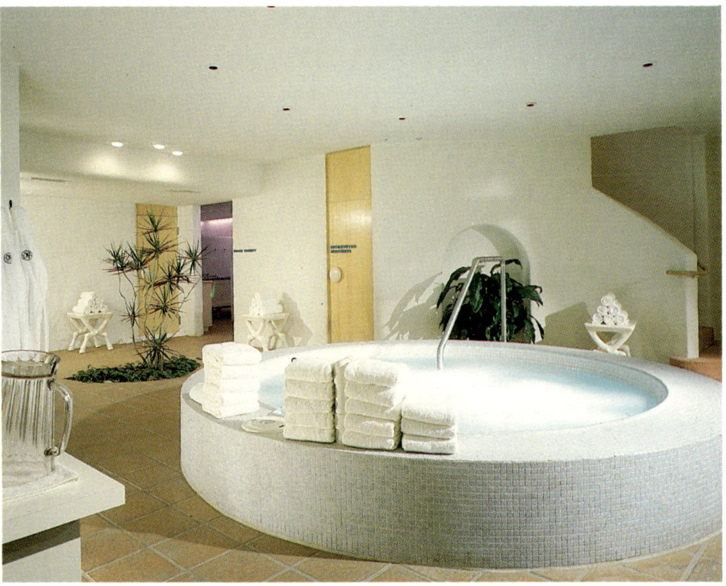

△ **A variety of exercise and therapy rooms radiate from the large circular whirlpool in this home gymnasium. White "goat leg" tables were designed by John Dickenson; Mexican terra-cotta tiles boast a slip-free finish.**

FITNESS SPA

This spacious health club was designed by Charles Swerz for the ultimate in fitness and relaxation. Created to accommodate both large and small groups, facilities were planned with adequacy and comfort in mind; a series of adjacent rooms are devoted to special activities such as tanning or exercising.

A palette of tile, stucco, and abundant natural light enhance the resortlike quality of the facility. A large circular whirlpool tub stands at the radial axis of all the adjacent rooms. Large enough to seat twelve people, the tub is surfaced in 1-inch square ceramic tiles and features an extra-wide ledge that doubles for seating. White laminate convenience counters are equipped with sinks, towels, and refrigerators, as well as drinking glasses and water pitchers. The floor is covered with Mexican terra-cotta tiles with a slip-resistant finish.

The adjoining exercise room features a selection of equipment with contact surfaces covered in turquoise leather. Included in the equipment profile are rowing machines, slant boards with ankle rollers, stationary ergometers, a trampoline, and a Gravity Guiding System. Stucco walls feature inset mirror panels to simulate architectural recesses; plexiglass roof panels flood the room with natural light.

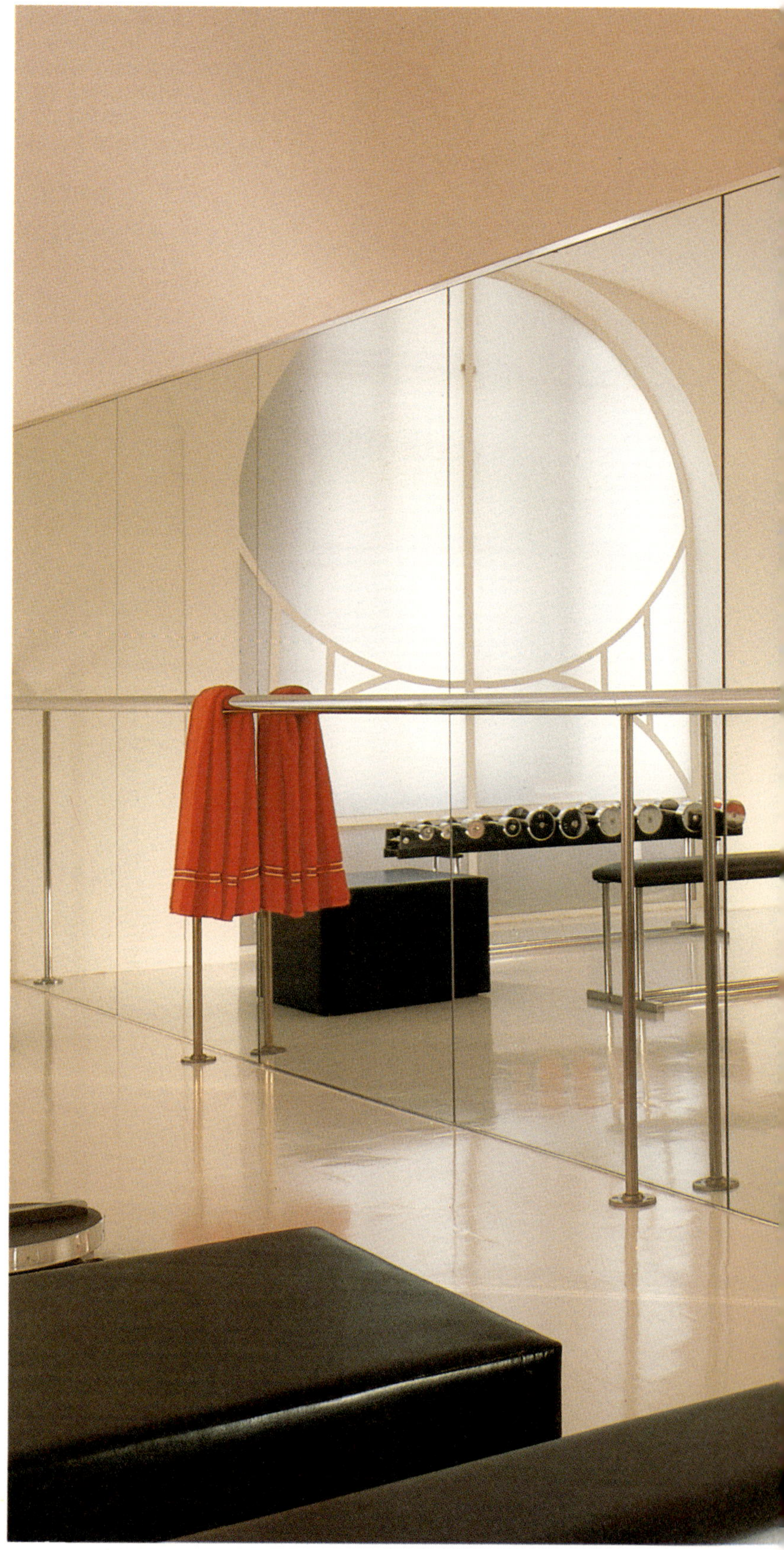

SUBURBAN SPACIOUS

David Snyder's design for this large suburban gym projects an air of sophisticated austerity. White vinyl floors and walls enhance the feeling of spaciousness, while floor-to-ceiling mirror panels allow clients to monitor their progress.

The gym features professionally styled equipment from Mac Levy ™. The five-station Torso Gym ™ is totally chrome-plated, with all contact surfaces covered in black leather. The solid-steel dumbbell set is also finished in polished chrome and is stored in its own freestanding rack. A leather upholstered exercise bench and custom-designed dancer's barre—running the full length of the mirrored wall—complete the equipment profile.

Designed in the neo-Gothic tradition, the arched frosted-glass window with decorative ironwork conceals an unappealing view.

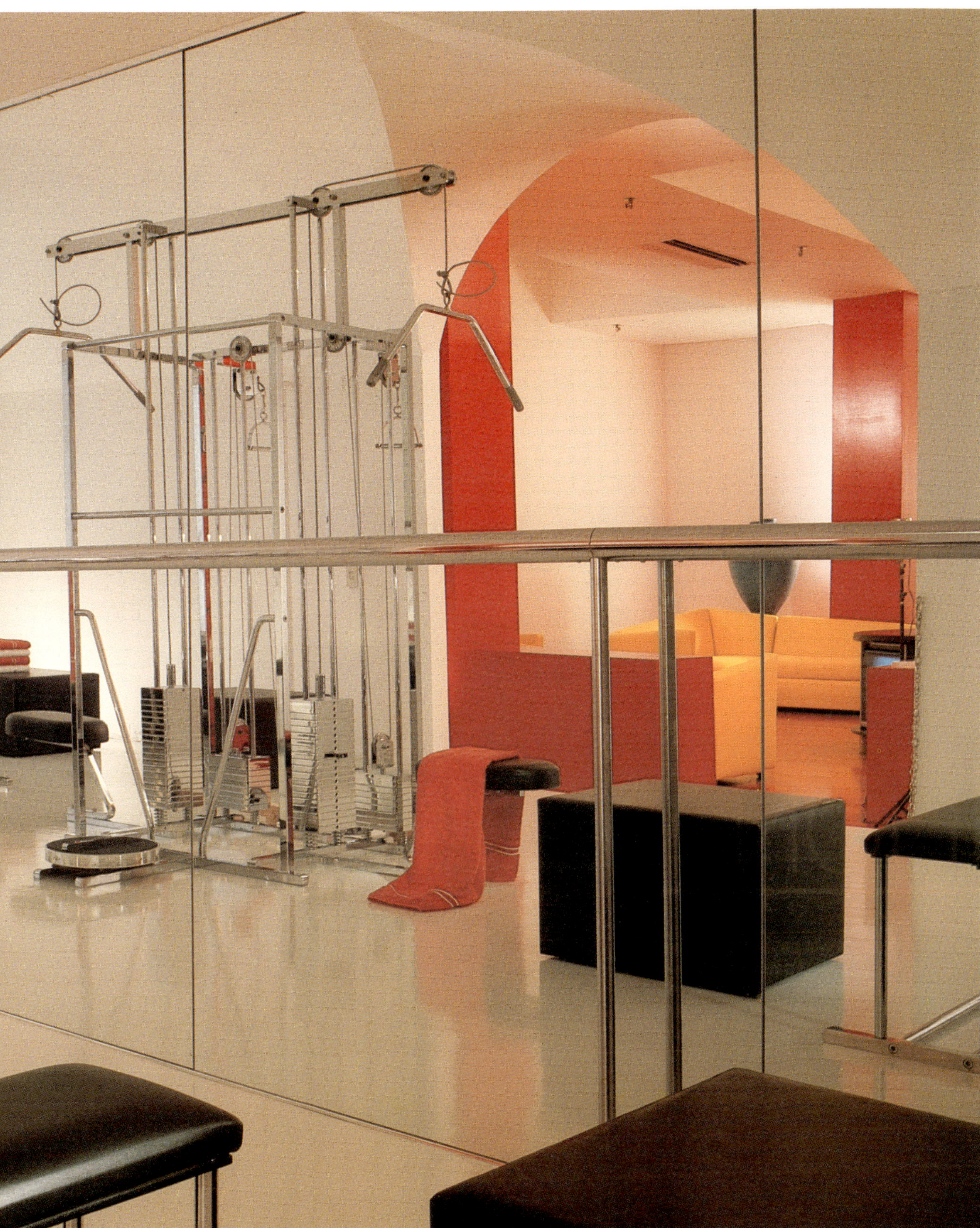

This spacious home gymnasium comfortably accommodates a variety of fitness equipment corrresponding to the client's preferred exercise circuit. Fabricated in brushed stainless steel, a custom-designed dancer's barre runs the full length of the gym's mirrored wall. All other equipment is from Mac Levy.

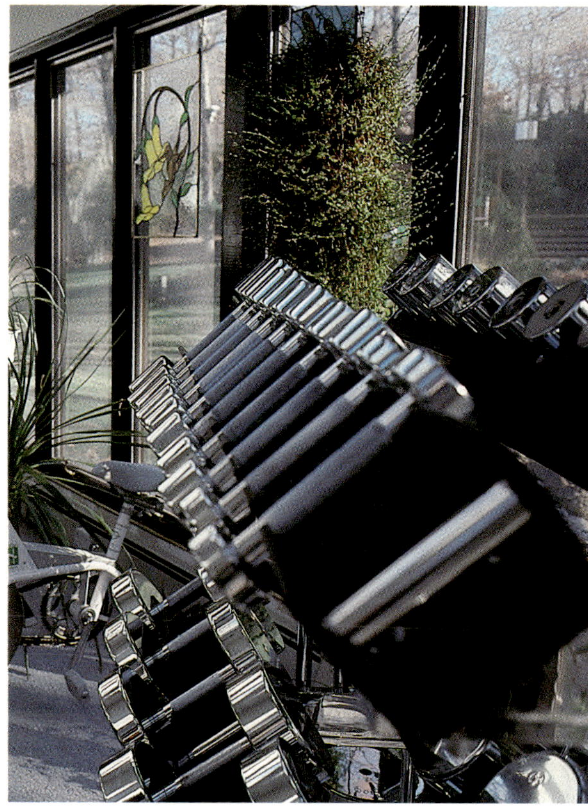

GARDEN PAVILION

Designed exclusively for exercise, this skylit pavilion borrowed its space from an existing but seldom used patio. Incorporating the view as a major decorative element, the designer used windows on three sides and a series of large skylights in the pitched roof. A chrome-plated multistation weightlifting machine and dumbbell set with stand were chosen as much for their looks as for their unobtrusive quality. For relaxing between routines, two plump sofas upholstered in removable cotton slipcovers are included in the design.

Mirror panels along the back wall reflect the garden view and allow the clients to watch their progress. Industrial-grade carpeting in dove-gray is softened by a thick foam padding for added comfort and resilience. A stationary ergometer and glass-enclosed shower complete the fitness amenities.

Large glass windows and skylights bring the restful garden view inside this exercise pavilion. Equipment was arranged according to the client's personal exercise circuit; overstuffed sofas are a welcome postexercise amenity.

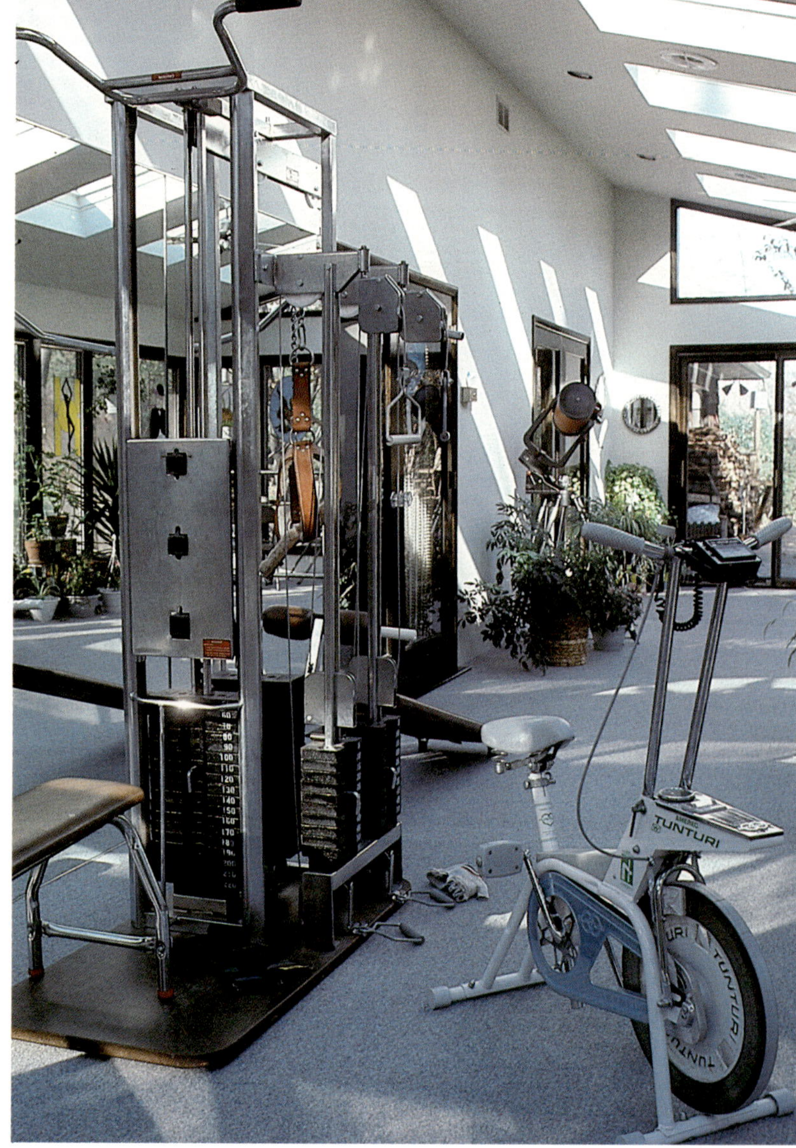

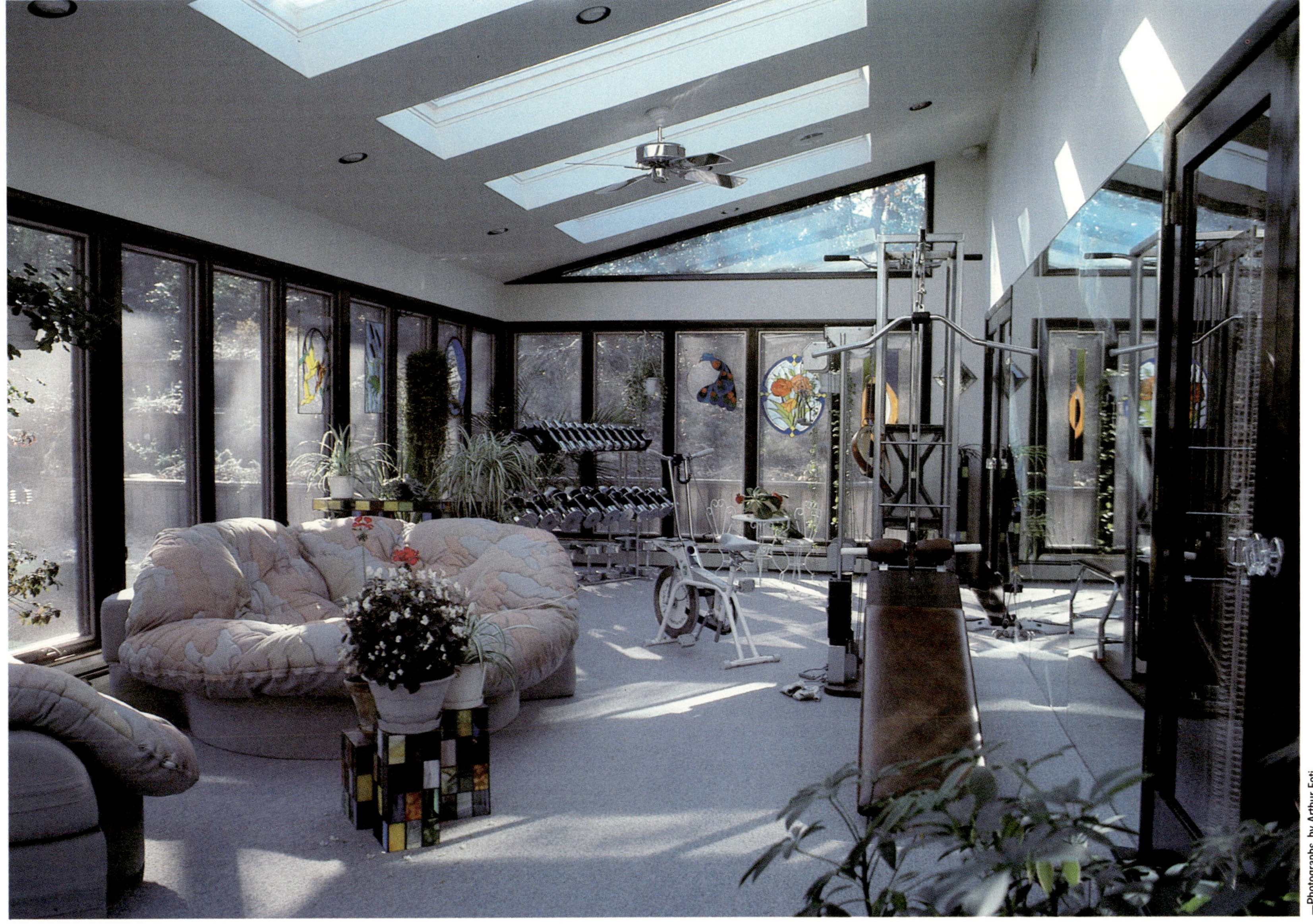

—Photographs by Arthur Foti

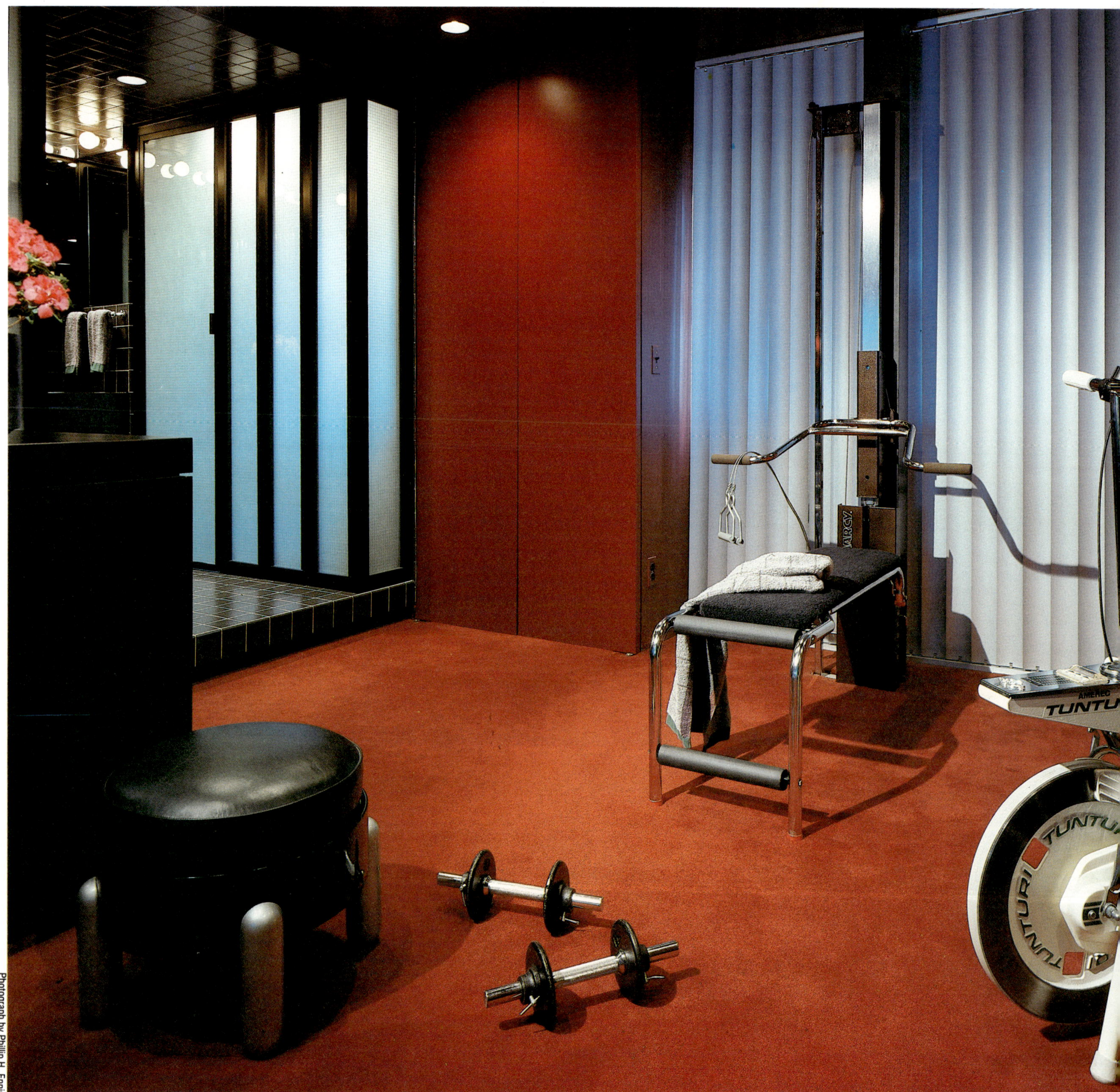

Photograph by Phillip H. Ennis

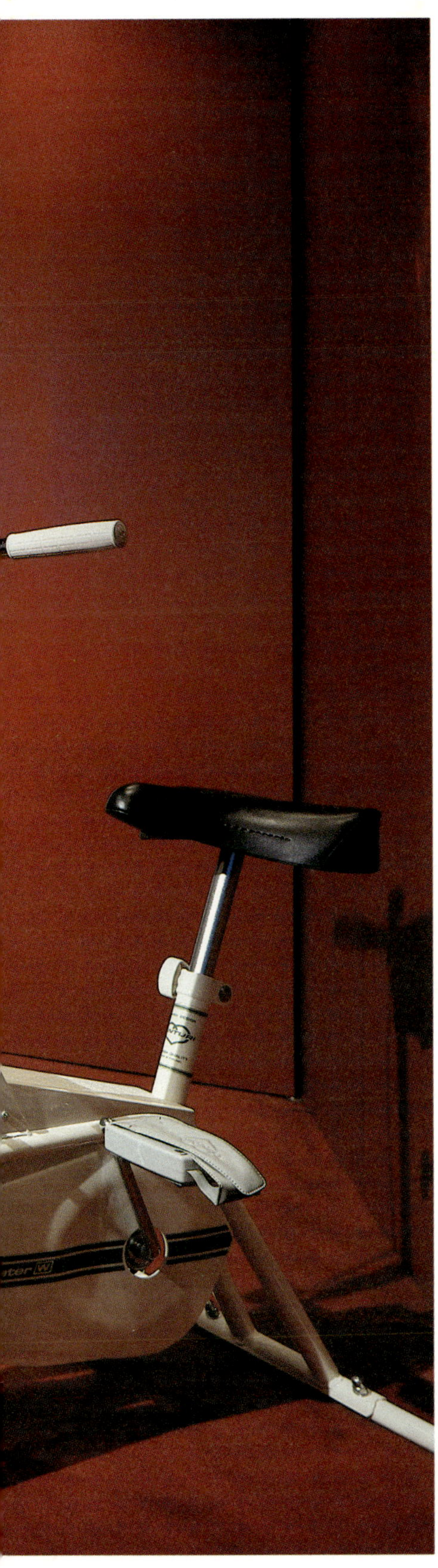

Multistation gym by Marcy, a Tunturi ergometer, and small free weights are conveniently placed beside the bath of this master bedroom. Rich coloration and an architectural wall treatment enhance the feeling of sensuous retreat; a small leather stool counterpoints the equipment's industrial honesty.

SENSUOUS RETREAT

Never one to succumb to the tedious conformity of lackluster minimalism, designer Eric Bernard enlivens his work with a touch of the unexpected. True to form, this mulberry-hued gymnasium/master bedroom reaffirms this tenet and elevates the concept of sensuous introspection to an art.

Bernard's strict architectural approach is mitigated by a palette of well-coordinated surface treatments and disarming color. Plush velvet carpeting, for example, establishes a visual dialogue between the slick lacquered walls and ceramic floor tiles of the master bath. Cosmetically deepened window wells enhance structural significance while recessed floodlights maintain the architectural integrity.

Furnishings were planned with deference to the fitness equipment—conveniently situated outside the master bath to facilitate a postexercise shower or sauna. The sauna enclosure itself also illustrates Bernard's unexpected sleight-of-hand: wire-impregnated glass panels were sandblasted for an opaque finish and framed by black anodized steel posts.

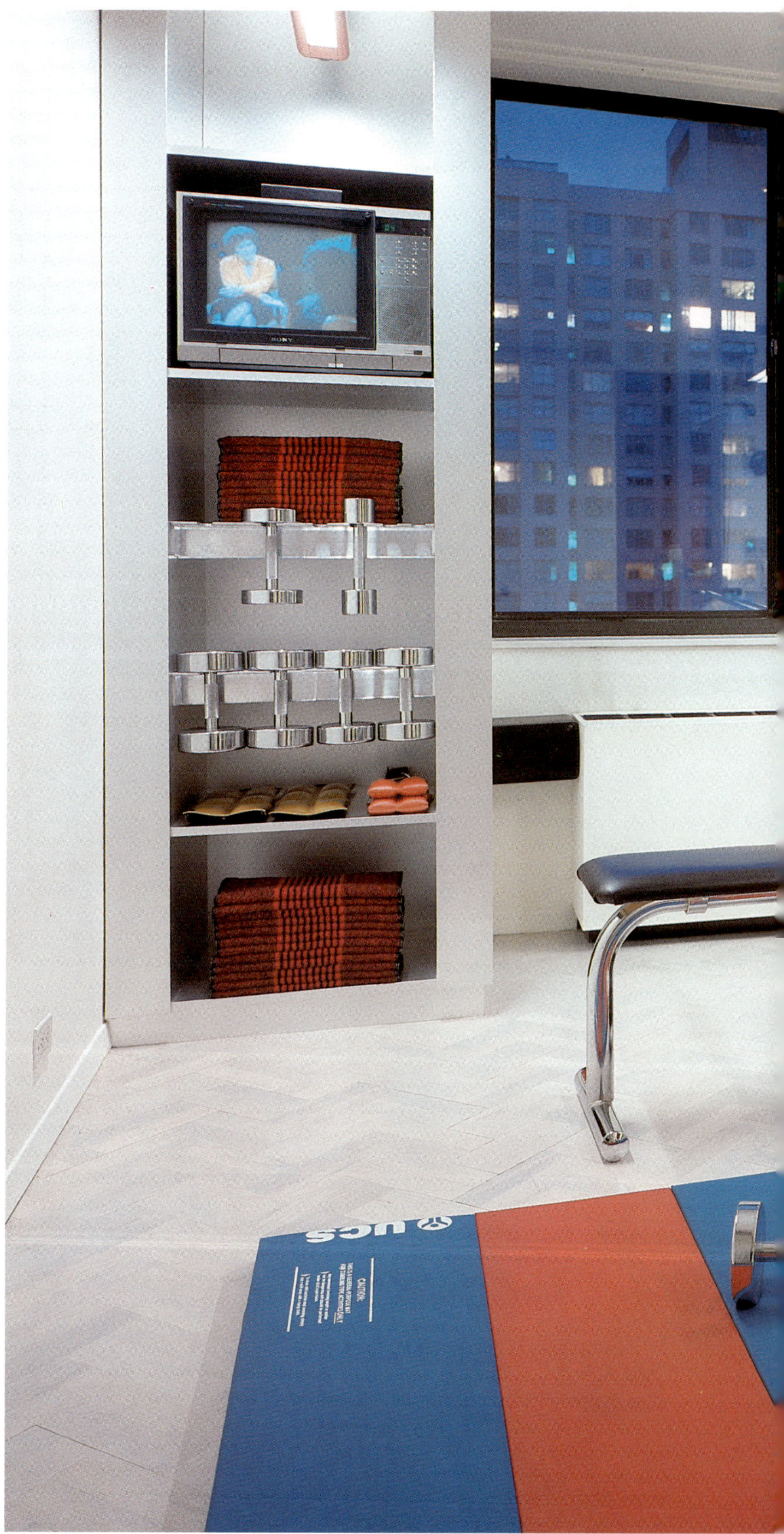

HONEST SENSIBILITY

For this New York home gymnasium, designer Maurice Bernstein shows a professional touch that is characteristically understated. There is no hint of the contrived or picturesque; in fact, the most recognized forms of effect are studiously, even puritanically, avoided. Instead Bernstein makes an argument for the virtues of clarity and intelligence. His sensibility combines uncorrupted forms and honest materials.

An all-white color palette, mirrored wall, and chromed weightlifting machine all lend a pristine elegance to the space. In keeping with the mood, Bernstein bleached and pickled the standard parquet flooring rather than specify a more conventional carpeted floor treatment. The only splash of color is, in fact, confined to the large exercise mat. Red, white, and blue never looked so good.

Bernstein designed a custom étagère/media unit in a corner beside the window. Notched cradles vertically organize the chromed dumbbells by size and weight while open shelves hold towels and accessories. The Sony monitor is used for diversion when using the stationary bicycle and for screening exercise videos.

White lacquered pendant fixtures—more commonly encountered in contract applications—hold fluorescent/incandescent lamps.

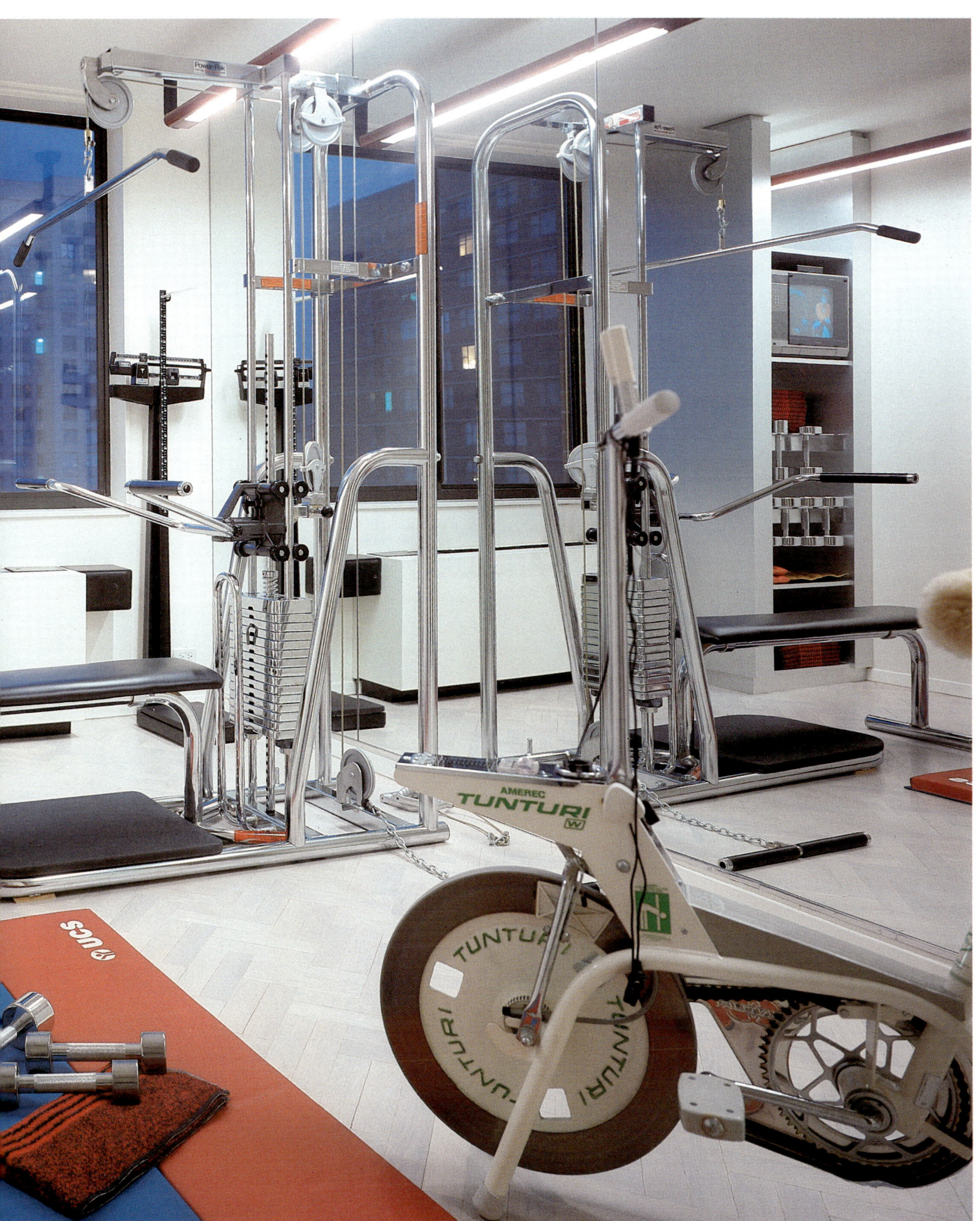

—Photograph by Phillip H. Ennis

A custom étagère/media cabinet easily organizes the client's free weights, towels, and accessories. The television monitor is used for both diversion and to screen exercise videos; standard parquet floors were bleached and pickled to achieve a lightly colored effect.

Since maintaining a healthy appearance is the name of the game for those in the public eye, it is no surprise to find a myriad of show business stars, would-be stars, and athletes following a regular program of exercise and balanced nutrition. Among such well-known fitness devotees are Tom Jones, Brooke Shields, Vidal Sassoon, and Virginio Ferrario.

CELEBRITY EXERSTYLE

—Photograph by Rex Features

Model/actress Brooke Shields's exercise routine focuses on figure maintenance and muscle tone. Avoiding the weightlifting machines, Shields prefers a strenuous routine of floor exercises, which she supplements with 3- and 6-pound dumbbells for added resistance. Leg raises for abdominal conditioning are performed with the aid of the Hip Flexor.

Photograph by Enrico Ferreli, Don Morley

Weightlifting is the passion of professional athlete Virginio Ferrario's exercise program. With an eye to muscular strength, tone, and definition, Ferrario prefers free weights to the weightlifting machines, always wearing a lifting belt as a safety measure. A ceiling-mounted punching bag helps develop footwork and timing while providing a good overall workout. Ferrario supplements this program with floor exercises such as push-ups, sit-ups and leg raises.

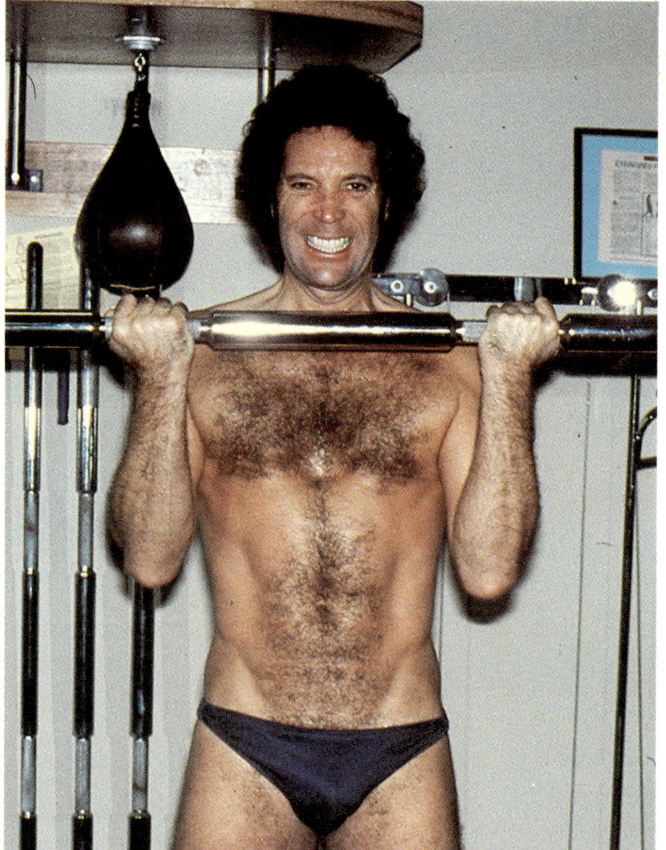

—Photograph by Rex Features

Singer/actor Tom Jones's △ exercise program is geared to muscle strength and weight control. The singer regularly trains with graduated barbells and augments his bending and stretching exercises with hand-held dumbbells. Bouts with a regulation punching bag satisfy Jones's pugilistic instincts.

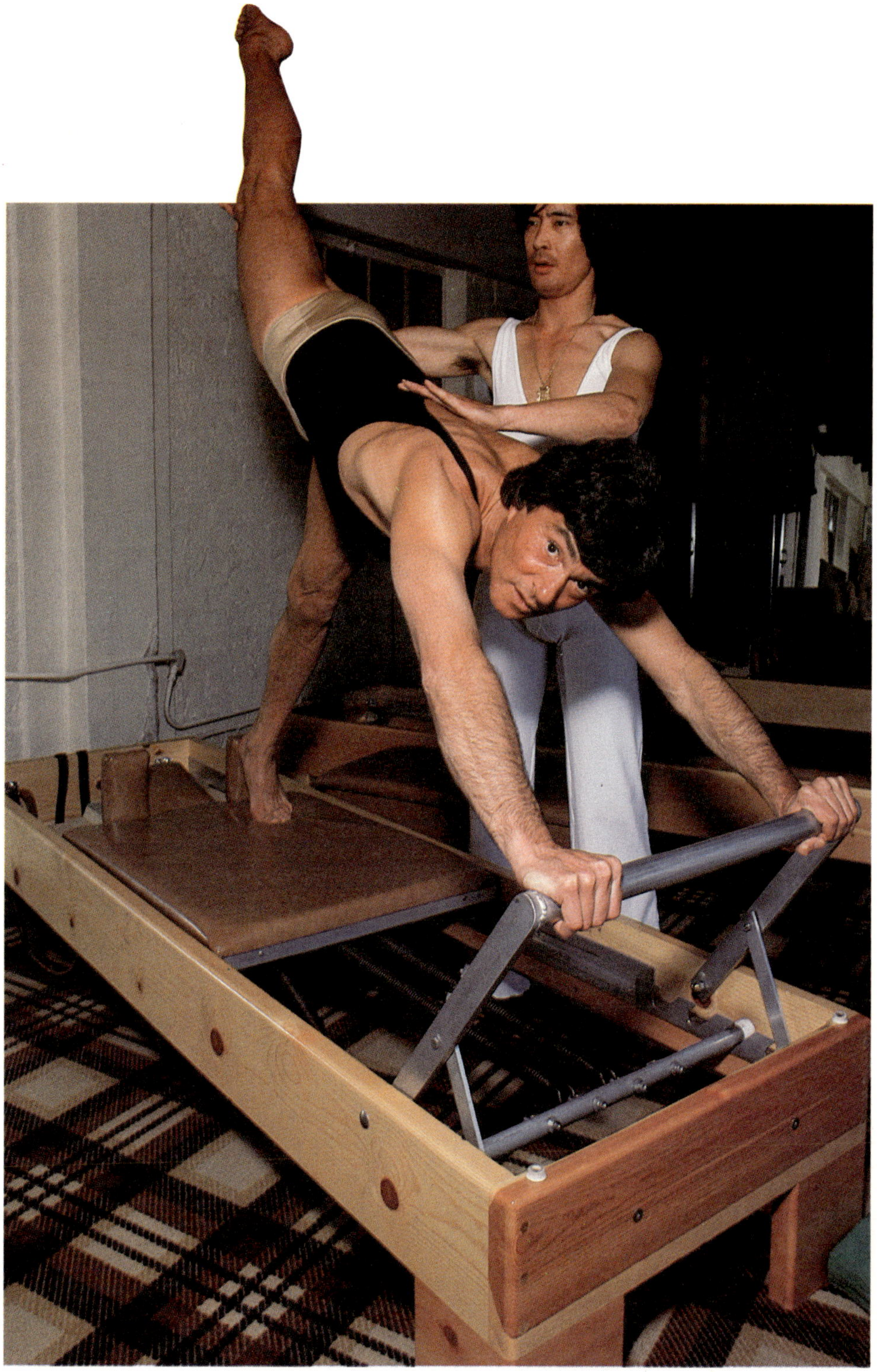

—Photograph by Rex Features

◁ Hair-care magnate Vidal Sassoon works out five times a week with his trainer in his own Beverly Hills gymnasium. Devoted to the Indian philosophy of physical harmony and well-being, Sassoon and his trainer have developed a program of stretching exercises and yoga including deep breathing and meditation.

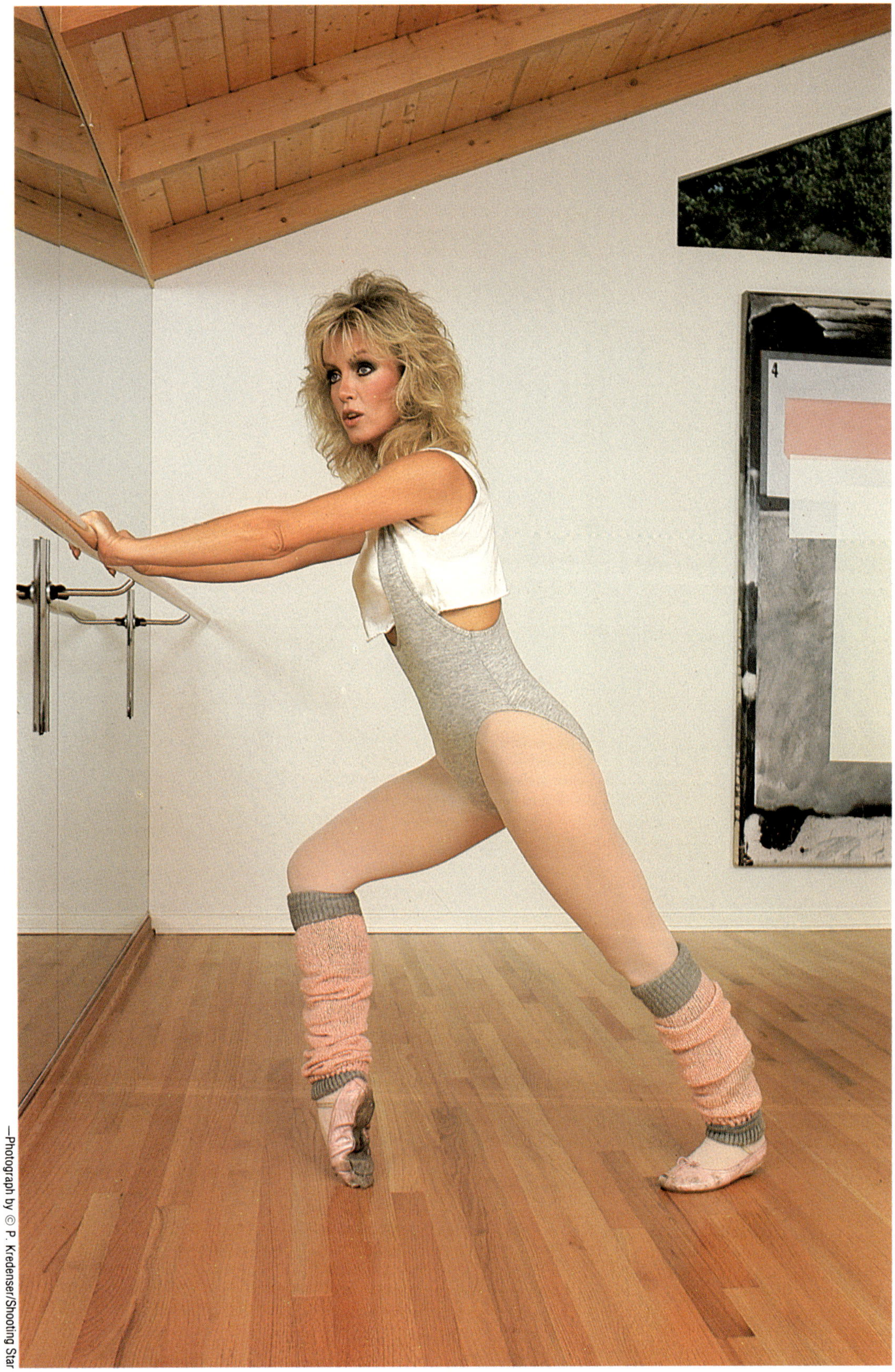

—Photograph by © P. Kredenser/Shooting Star

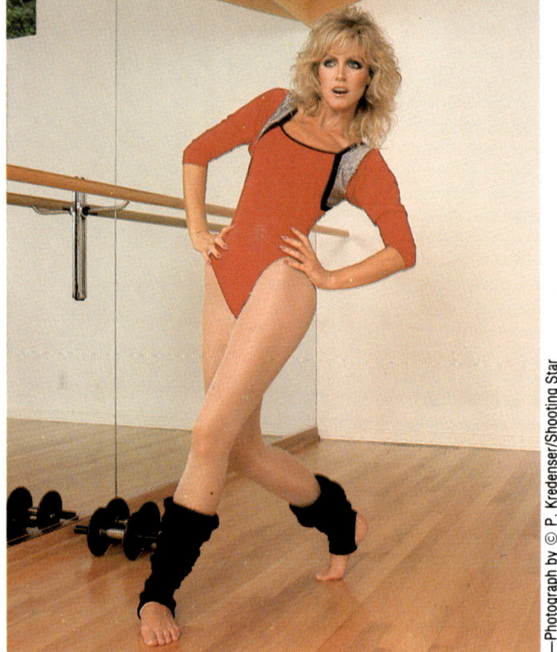

—Photograph by © P. Kredenser/Shooting Star

The mainstay of actress Donna Mills's exercise program is her home dance studio. A recent addition to her California home, the architect-designed wing features a timber-beamed cathedral ceiling, oversized skylights, and the mandatory dancer's barre. Floor-to-ceiling mirror panels allow Mills to chart her progress while favorite pieces from an extensive art collection add a note of warmth to the otherwise bare space.

Updating a repertoire of ballet exercises with her own limbering-up moves, the dancer's barre is Mills's favorite workout aid. Preferring the simple approach to conditioning, Mills eschews the more "advanced" equipment and supplements her routines with floor work on an exercise mat.

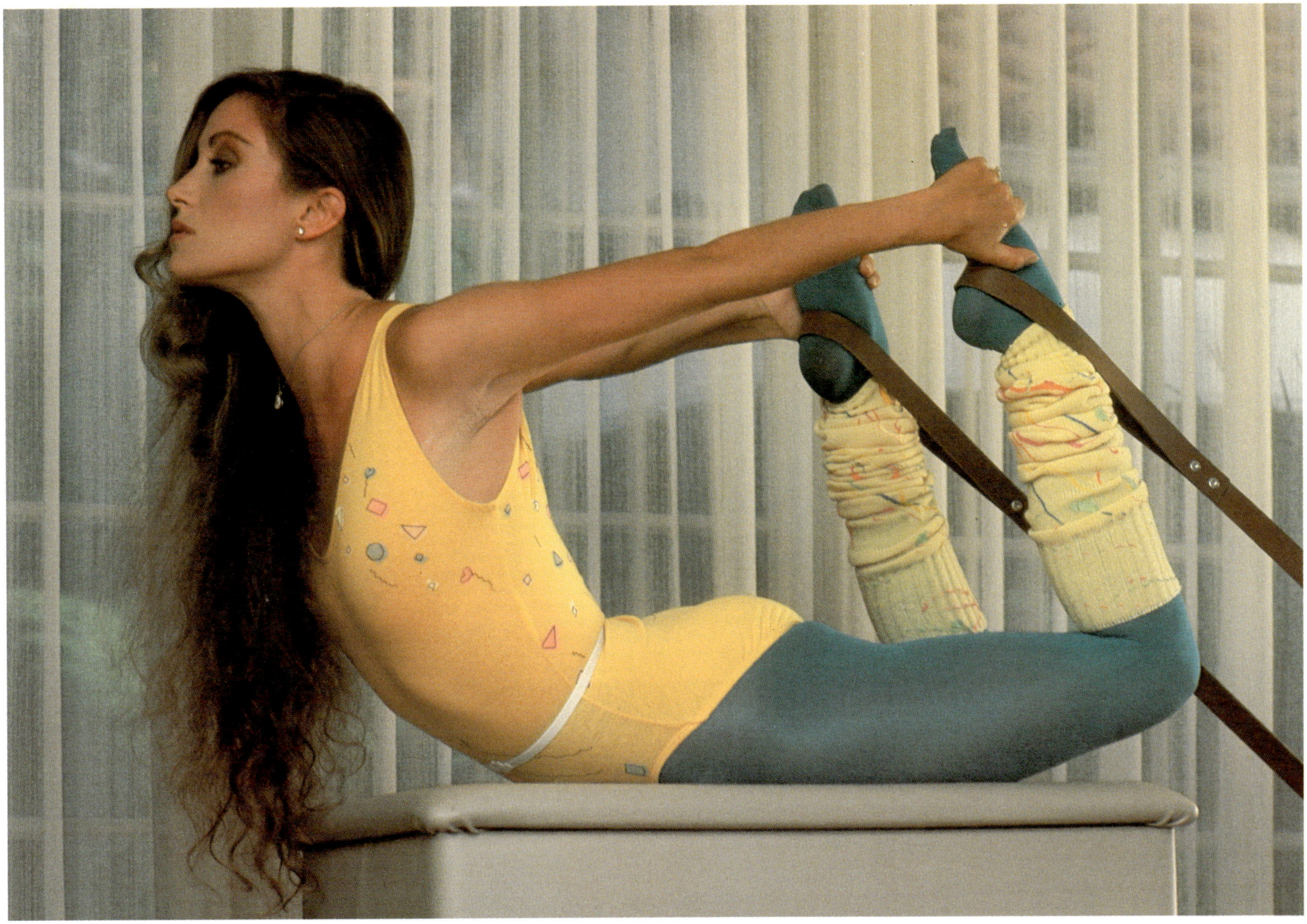

—Photographs by © Yoram Kahana

Actress Jane Seymour is committed to a program of figure maintenance with daily workouts. A long-time exercise aficionada, Seymour has been training at Wanda Bouvier's fitness studio since 1977. As recently as eighteen months ago, however, Seymour purchased a new exercise machine, which she has incorporated into her daily routine. Called The Body Balance, this sophisticated exercise table was invented by Wanda Bouvier to accommodate numerous exercises and stretching positions.

Seymour's program consists of

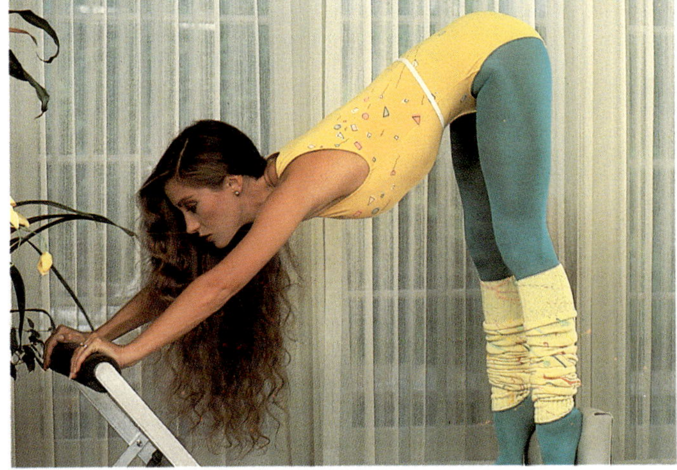

one hour on the machine supplemented by extensive floor work. The machine has also proven to be a motivator of sorts—the user starts out with the easiest moves and works at his or her own pace up to the more difficult ones. The "V" stomach pull, for example, is the most basic move, while the arabesque is very advanced.

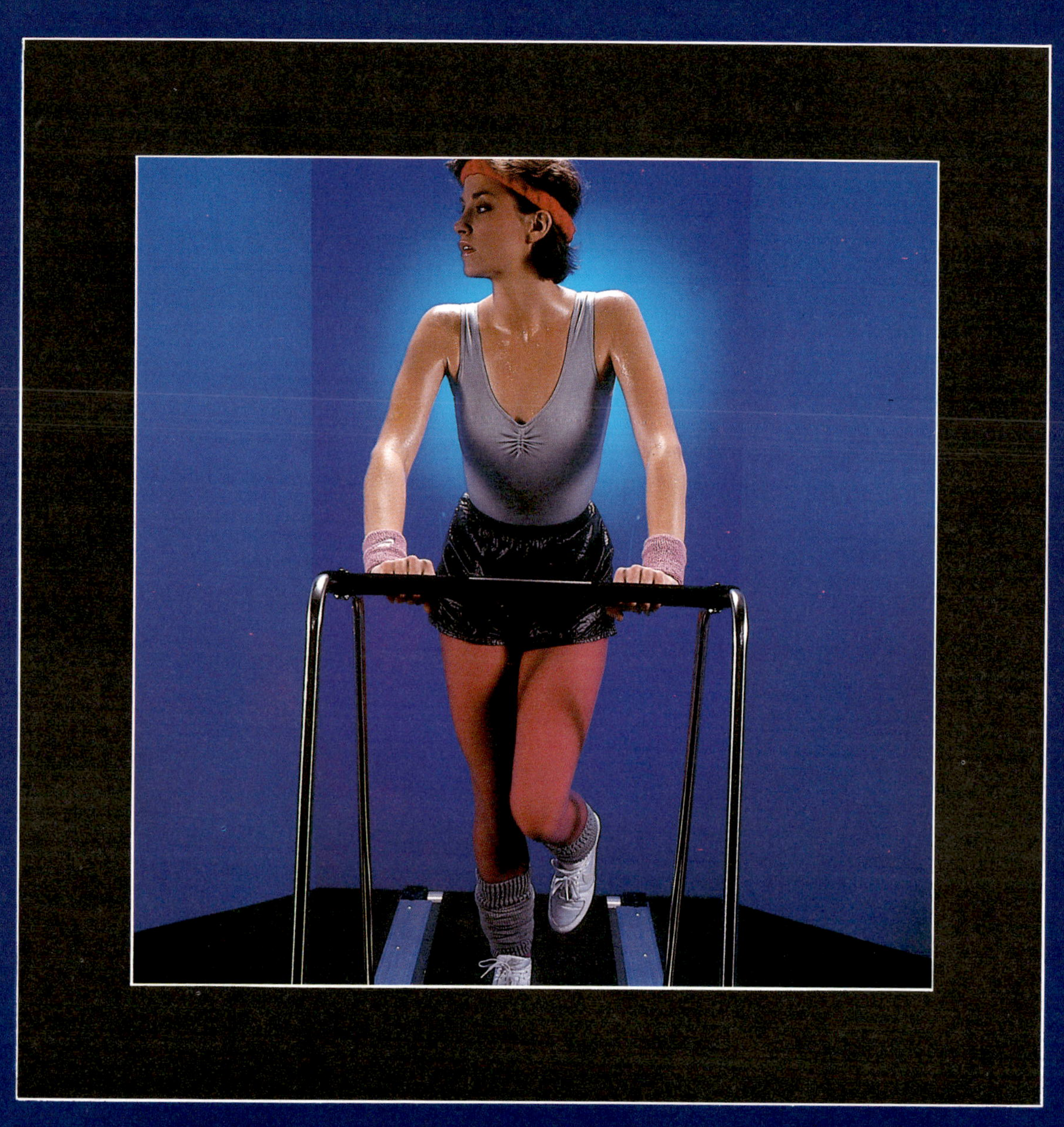

CHAPTER THREE

HEALTH AND FITNESS PORTFOLIO

FREDERICK C. HATFIELD, Ph.D.
Editor-in-Chief, *Sports Fitness* magazine

Picture this scenario. You walk into a health club for the first time in your life, driven there by a new awareness of the importance of fitness. You feel you don't belong there, but you go anyway. You are confronted by all the things you dreaded over a lifetime of inactivity: sweating, straining, heavy breathing. Even people drinking healthy stuff like carrot juice or guava nectar.

But you have made up your mind that no matter what, you'll persevere—at least until you shed some twenty pounds of ugly fat and flatten your tummy enough to deserve a few sideward glances while walking along the pavement. So in you go, determined but somewhat frightened and confused by the incredible array of strange noises and space-age contraptions.

"I hope the instructor knows what he's doing," you mutter to yourself from between clenched teeth. "This place reminds me of a Star Wars torture chamber!"

Happily, the instructor does know. And a few short months later, you walk out of the gym the proud owner of a renovated body—and outlook.

What went on in there? What could cause such a metamorphosis in your appearance and spirit? Believe me, there's nothing magical about becoming fit. The marriage of science with technology has, over the past few years, produced a number of machines and techniques that make the task of reshaping the human body child's play. And the process can be fun besides!

This chapter will spotlight the body—how it works, how it responds to exercise, and which machines work best for each part of the body.

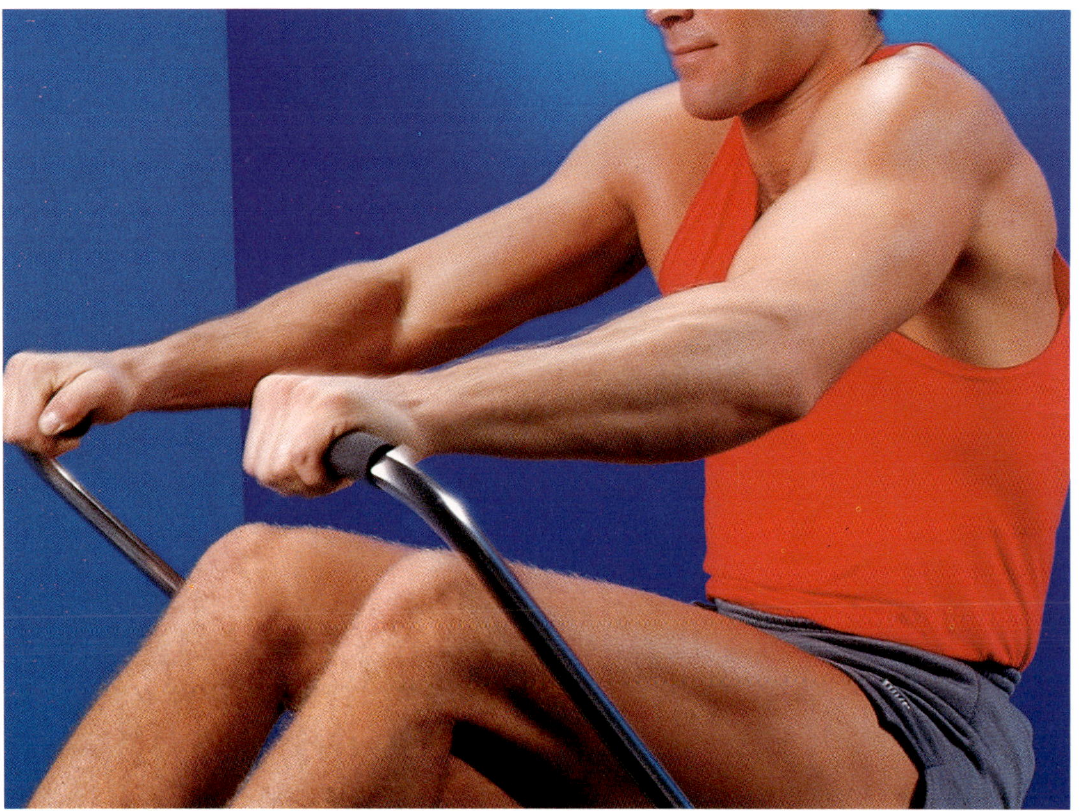

Your Body: How It Works

Once you've made the commitment to exercise, whether at a health club or in your home, you will have to invest time and money in either suitable home equipment or a membership to a suitable health club. Once that's taken care of, you'll have to decide on a training program that will allow you to achieve your fitness goals with the least amount of wasted time and energy.

Understanding how your body works and how it responds to the different forms of fitness technology will enable you to choose home equipment or gym facilities more knowledgeably. And the more you know about something, the more likely you are to enjoy it. It is no accident that the fitness boom has not subsided: Now that people are becoming more sophisticated in their knowledge of their bodies and the effect various kinds of fitness equipment have on their bodies, the entire process has become more enjoyable to them. The fitness movement is here to stay.

Before you develop a fitness program, you should know what scientists call the *principles of conditioning*. They center on the well-known law that in order for muscles to become stronger, more toned, bigger, or more enduring they have to be *stressed*. Stress is the most important requirement of any kind of fitness program, whether you're a professional athlete, a dancer, a weekend warrior, or a housekeeper interested in getting in shape.

What kind of stress do you need? How much? How often? That's what the principles of conditioning are all about.

- To increase the strength, size, or endurance of your muscles, you must stress them *more than they're used to*.
- As you grow stronger, bigger, or more enduring, you must continue to *increase the stress*.
- *Strength* (the ability to apply force) is best increased by applying between 75% and 85% of your maximum force when exercising with weights or machines.
- *Muscle strength* is best increased when you use a variety of stress levels (ranging between 50% and 85%) in your training program.
- *Muscle endurance* (the ability to do sustained work) is improved most efficiently when your training load is between 50% and 75% of your maximum force.
- The quality of overload—making the muscles work harder than they're used to—is improved by applying stress through the full range of movement in any given exercise.
- To improve or maintain joint flexibility, adaptive stress should be applied to *all* the muscles surrounding a joint—never only those on one side.
- To improve *power* (explosive, fast movement) each movement should be completed as quickly as possible, and the best level of stress is between 65% and 80% of your maximum force.
- The best way to improve the strength, size, endurance, or power of a muscle is to find an exercise that effectively *isolates* its action from that of surrounding muscles.
- The best way to improve a sport *skill,* aside from practicing it, is to overload *specific movement patterns* used in that skill *as well as* to overload the *individual muscles* used in that skill.

There are a few more basic principles that could be listed, but those listed are the most important ones to remember. In fact, these are the ones to consider when choosing a health club or choosing weight training equipment for your home gym. They are also the ones that you will have to apply when faced with the task of deciding on the best exercises for you.

Several questions are raised by the above list of basic principles. How do I determine what each of my muscle's *maximum force* ability is? How many *repetitions* of each exercise should I do? *How many exercises* should I do at each training session? *What is the best equipment* for me to use? How should I *breathe* when exercising? And, what about *warming up* and *cooling down*?

These questions will be answered in turn. They, together with the principles of conditioning listed above, will guide you in your efforts to achieve fitness in the most efficient and effective way possible.

Determining Your Maximum Force

Your maximum force capability is determined by how much weight each muscle can move through its range of movement for a single repetition. Competitive weightlifters and powerlifters are the only people who should ever truly test themselves this way. You don't have to, and you shouldn't. It's dangerous.

The chart below will guide you instead. For example, when you're able to do ten repetitions with a weight in any exercise, you're probably using in the neighborhood of 80% of your muscle force capability to do so. Or, if you're only able to do five repetitions before your muscles become too fatigued to go any farther, you're using approximately 90% of your total strength. The chart is accurate for most people, so don't even bother trying to determine your maximum strength by lifting as much as you can at one time. Simply use the chart and then approximate from it your muscles' total strength.

A SUMMARY OF THE METHODS OF WEIGHT TRAINING FOR VARIOUS OBJECTIVES

Variable	Power	Strength	Local Muscular Endurance	Size
SETS	4–6	4–6	Maximum	4–6
REPETITIONS	3–8	3–8	25–40	Varies
METHOD	Explosive using compensatory acceleration	Moderate cadence	Slow, continuous cadence	Varies
REST INTERVALS	Short pause with relaxation between reps and 2–6 minutes between sets	Short pause with relaxation between reps and 2–6 minutes between sets	Allow heart rate to return to manageable level between sets	Varies

*Adapted from Hatfield, F.C. *Complete Guide to Power Training,* Fitness Systems, 1983. Used by permission.

How Many Repetitions and Sets Should I Do?

A *repetition* is one complete movement—with a barbell or weight machine, for example. A *set* is a group of repetitions. There is a method for determining the proper number of repetitions and sets you should do, and it depends on what your training goals are.

Take another look at the objectives chart. You will see that for each goal (power, size, strength, or endurance) there is a range of repetitions noted. These guidelines are scientifically determined by looking at the changes that occur inside a muscle cell after several weeks of training in a certain way.

You will notice that numerous repetitions with a light weight produce muscle changes relating to endurance, whereas fewer repetitions with a heavier weight produce stronger muscles. Bodybuilding, which concentrates on muscle size, is most effectively accomplished by a variety of repetition schemes, in an effort to affect a number of cellular changes rather than just one.

When your muscles become too fatigued to accomplish another set at the intensity level noted on the chart, you have done the right number of sets. Typically, you will be able to perform 3–5 sets before you become too fatigued to do another while maintaining the proper level of intensity (that is, the proper percentage of your maximum).

You should rest for approximately 3–5 minutes between sets to allow your muscles to recover a bit and to allow your heart rate to come back down to a manageable level.

For the first few weeks of exercising, you

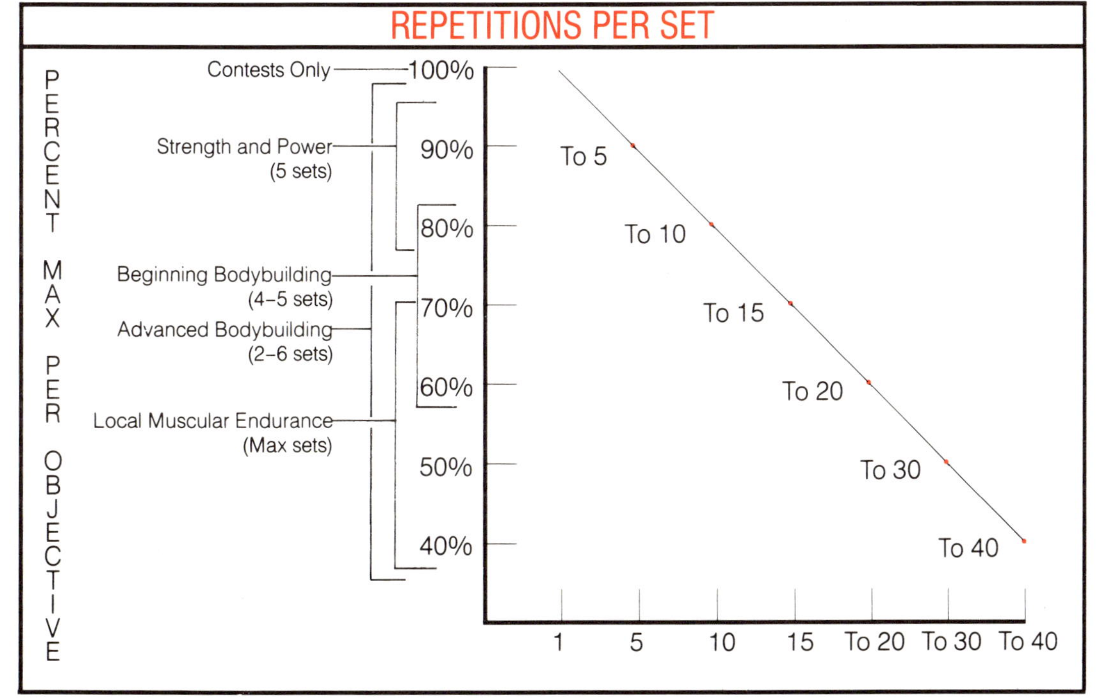

should not try to achieve the guidelines for repetitions and sets listed in the chart. Instead, work into it slowly, performing only a bit more than what you were used to doing. Soon you will be able to perform at maximum effectiveness—don't rush it!

Choosing the Proper Exercises

Stand in front of a mirror and give your physique a critical look. Arms too small? Abdominal muscles loose and bulging? Chest flat? Skinny legs? Shoulders stooped and rounded?

Or, if you're an athlete, critically evaluate your body in relation to a particular sport's physical requirements. Need explosive legs? Enduring arms? Strength for lifting, throwing, jumping, or swinging a bat?

When you have listed all of your conditioning goals, you have, in effect, mapped out the two important guides in determining what exercises to do. First, you have given yourself a guide for picking the proper number of repetitions and sets to do (for strength, power, endurance, or size); and second, you have identified the muscles you want to work on.

But knowing which muscle and which exercise isn't enough. You must also be able to choose which machine or implement to use in order to achieve your goal most efficiently. Guidelines for machine selection are listed later in this chapter. There are virtually dozens of machines and exercise apparatuses from which to choose, and the selection process can be quite confusing!

When deciding on the exercises you need in order to reach your fitness or conditioning goals, you must remember that each exercise will cause you to become a bit more fatigued. You will not be able to do more than approximately ten exercises in any given workout because your fatigue level will not allow it. So, choose your exercises wisely, making sure that each will deliver maximum results. One or 2 exercises per body part and 10 exercises per workout are sufficient.

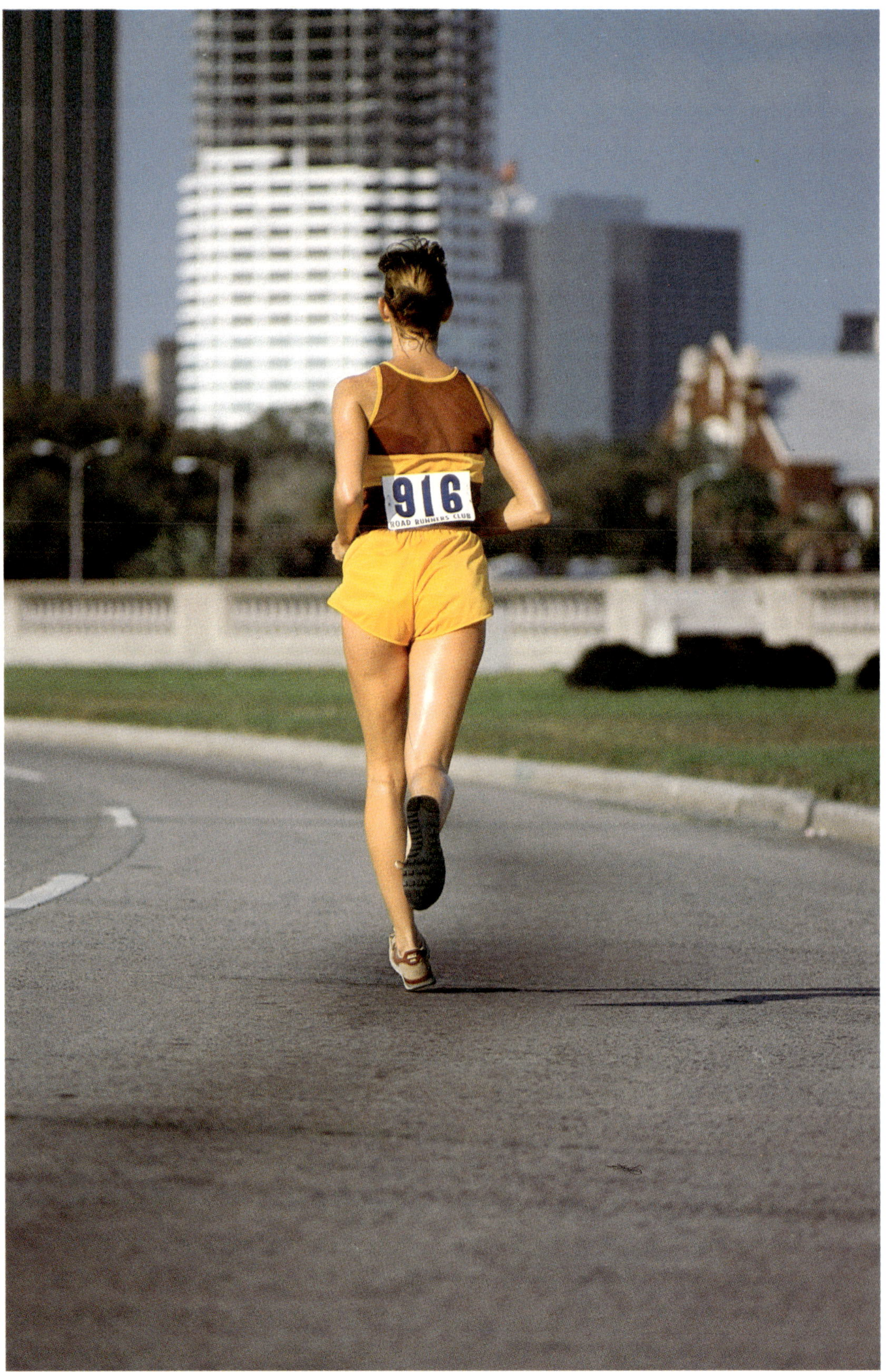

Whether you run for fitness or to compete, you'll need to prepare your body beforehand with "foundation" training to prevent unnecessary injuries.

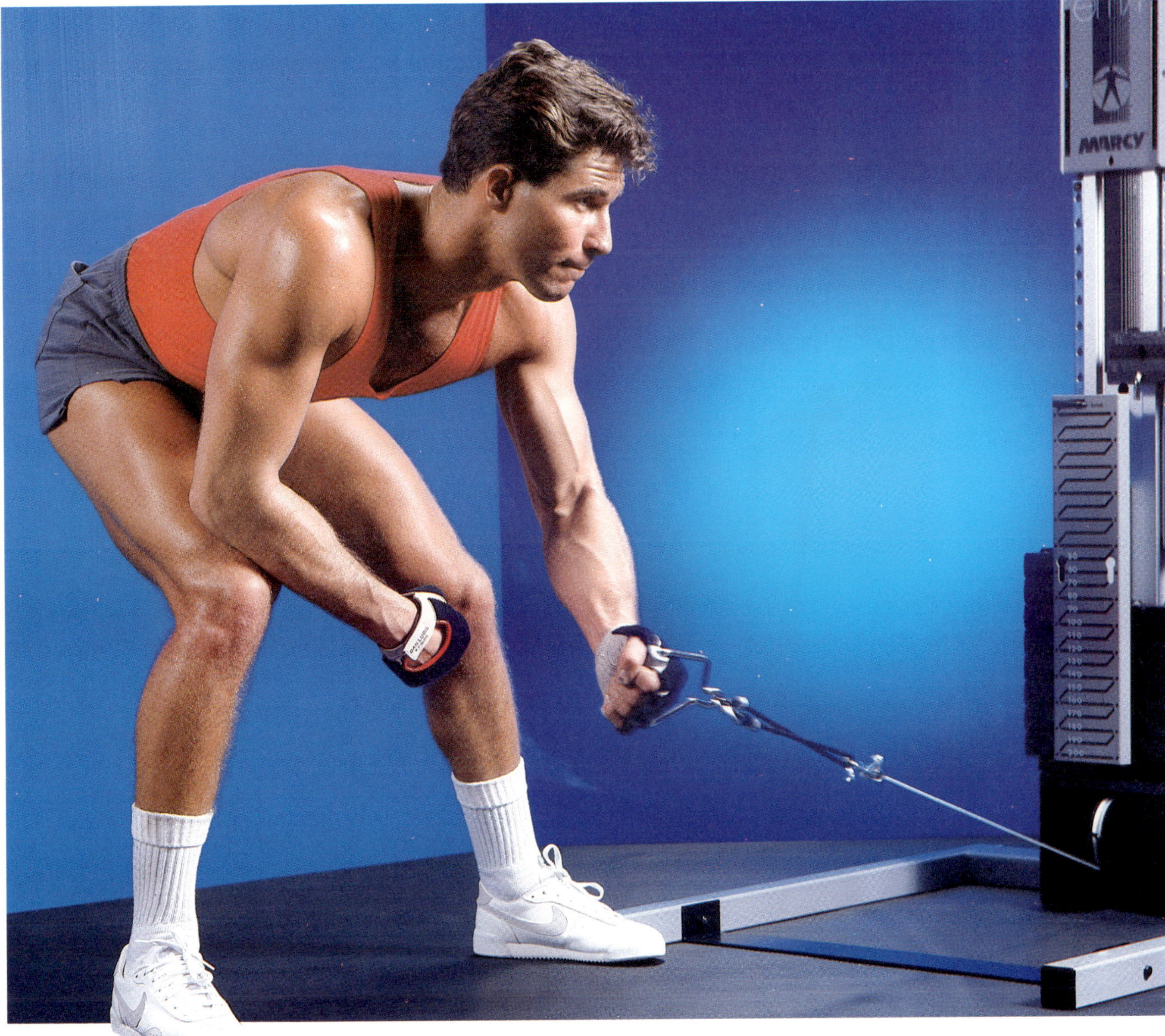

Cables attached to weight stacks provide great versatility in exercise selection. With this low pulley, you can stress all the major muscles of the body.

How Often Should I Work Out?

Remember the old saying, "Fools rush in where wise men fear to tread"? Don't rush into a training program determined to get instantaneous results. Working out too often and too hard will not help you reach your goals any faster; in fact, it may just slow you down or discourage you altogether. Sore or injured muscles and joints are no joke! And training too hard or too often is the most certain way of causing them. At the risk of boring you with old sayings, here's a final one: "Slow and steady wins the race."

The time it takes for your muscles to recuperate between workouts can vary, depending on 1) muscle size (larger muscles take longer), 2) age (older people recover more slowly), 3) training intensity (heavy training for strength requires longer recuperation time than does lighter training for endurance), and 4) fitness level (the fitter you are the shorter the recovery time necessary between workouts).

On the average, you should be able to train each muscle three times per week. Monday, Wednesday, and Friday is the most typical training schedule. If you have more than ten exercises to accomplish, you may want to use a *split routine,* which requires daily workouts.

For example, a typical split may look like this:

MONDAY WEDNESDAY FRIDAY	TUESDAY THURSDAY SATURDAY
chest, shoulders, upper arms, forearms, upper back	lower back, sides, abdominals, hips, thighs, lower legs

Flexibility and Warming Up

Every workout should be preceded and followed by flexibility and warm-up/cool-down exercises. Stretching and general warming up exercises prepare your muscles for a strenuous workout; stretching and cooling down after your workout help prevent postexercise muscle soreness and allow your heart rate to return to normal slowly.

Here is a great way to conduct your workout sessions:

STRETCHING:
Your shoulders, spine, and hip joints are the ones most vulnerable to injury from overexertion. Slowly stretch the muscles associated with these joints, avoiding jerky or bouncing movements. Each muscle should be stretched for about 1 minute, but not so much that you feel pain. A complete stretching session should last for about 10 minutes.

WARMING UP:
A slow jog around the gym or jogging in place for about 4 or 5 minutes will gear your body up for your weight training workout by raising your overall body temperature a degree or two. Another great warm-up exercise is skipping rope. Before performing each weight training exercise, you should also warm up the specific muscle(s) that will be stressed during the exercise by performing a set or two with extremely light weights.

EXERCISE SESSION:
After thoroughly stretching and warming up, perform your planned workout.

COOL-DOWN:
After working out, jog in place or around the gym for 2 or 3 minutes. Follow the short jog with a minute of rapid walking. This will allow your heart rate to return to normal gradually, thereby preventing "blood pooling" in any specific muscle group.

STRETCHING:
A brief session of stretching following your workout helps to prevent undue muscle soreness from heavy training.

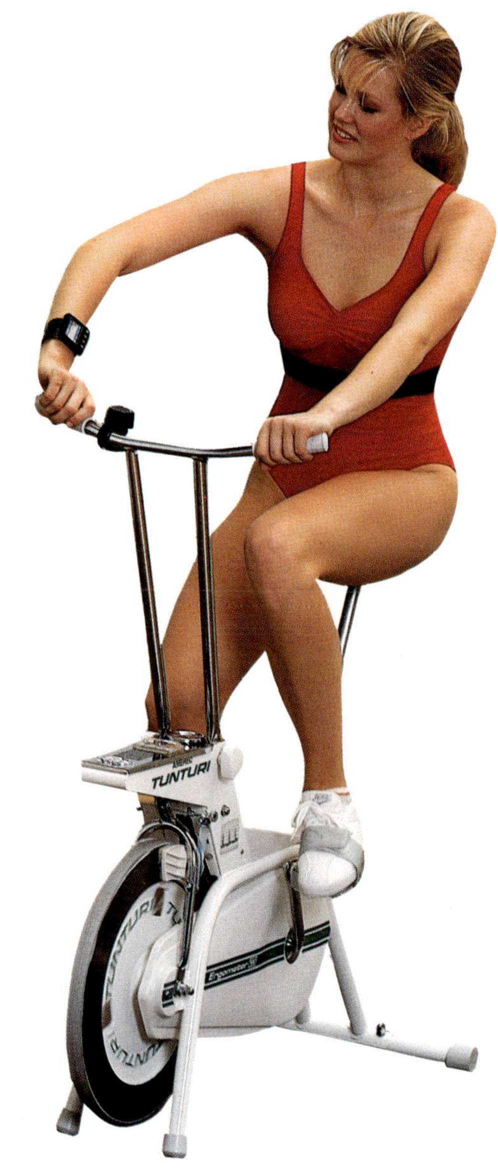

BREATHING:
If you hold your breath during a particularly heavy lift, you may run the risk of shutting down blood flow to the brain. This can cause *anoxia,* a shortage of oxygen in the brain. So, a simple rule of thumb while exercising is *don't hold your breath for long periods.*

Most experts agree that you should exhale when lifting the weight and inhale while lowering the weight or at the top of the lift. This is often difficult, however, because the heavy weight causes pressure to build up in the lungs and it may be difficult to control your breathing pattern. Besides, the pressure in your lungs helps to stabilize your chest and shoulder muscles so that they can more easily exert maximum force.

So, it is sometimes advisable to hold your breath for a short period during the exercise—during the phase of the lift when you are just beginning to contract the muscles for the lift. The added stability afforded by thoracic pressure will make the lift a bit easier. On the way up, however, begin to exhale to release the pressure.

During light sets in which 10 or more repetitions are being performed, breathing rarely becomes a problem. Simply breathe normally—do what comes naturally. Thoracic pressure rarely becomes a problem when lighter weights are used.

The Four Technologies of Fitness Machines

Some sociologists believe that the fitness boom is a backlash resulting from the inactivity forced on modern man by the age of technology. People *want* to be fit and are doing so in increasing numbers throughout the world. It's a bit ironic then, that the fitness industry is itself becoming more and more "high tech" and that the applications of technology are actually making it easier for us to get back in shape!

In prehistoric days, cavemen stayed strong by lifting rocks. The early pioneers lifted logs. Today, necessities of life do not control how or whether we remain fit. It is up to us to choose whether to do so and science can offer us the tools with which to do so effectively. The denizens of the drawing board, those biomechanicians who have our best interests at heart, have produced four different technologies from which we can choose to ward off the devastating effects of inactivity that our lifestyles have forced on us.

Let's return now to the first time you ever walked into the health club. Remember? You probably heard noises from chains clanking over pear-shaped sprockets, air releasing from valves, the squishing of fluid being forced through tiny apertures, and—most noticeable of all—the clang of heavy iron hitting the floor. A cornucopia of biotechnology! Fascinating as it was, you probably hoped that someone would put you on the one that hurt least.

Let's look at the four basic forms of fitness equipment that the technocrats who rule the fitness marketplace have devised.

CONSTANT RESISTANCE DEVICES

The term *constant resistance* means that a weight (resistance) does not increase or decrease during the course of exercise. The resistance remains constant from the beginning of an exercise movement to the completion of it.

No matter how many times you lift a barbell or dumbbell, the weight remains the same. When you lift a weight attached to a cable and pulley system, the weight remains the same too, provided the pulley is round rather than elliptical.

This form of weight training (or *resistance* training) has one major drawback: It doesn't correct for changes in musculoskeletal leverage that occur during an exercise movement. (When you lift a weight your leverage changes during the joint movement.) For example, when you perform a deep-knee bend, or a squat, with a barbell resting on your shoulders, the amount of muscular force you have to exert near the bottom of the squat movement is far more than the force near the top of the movement. The reason for this is that the closer to the erect standing position you come, the more your musculoskeletal leverage improves. The improved leverage means that you don't have to work as hard during the easy phase of the movement and therefore benefit somewhat less than you do during the hard phase. Remember the most important law of conditioning: Your muscles need stress to grow bigger, stronger, or more enduring. With some of the beneficial stress gone, the exercise is a bit less effective than it might be.

However, constant resistance exercises also have their advantages. Many fitness scientists believe that constant resistance training is more natural and therefore more effective in the long run. In other words, the changes in musculoskeletal leverage during the movement of an exercise conform to the way the human body works, so that exercising that way will help you achieve better results.

As we shall see, however, there are also those who believe that we can improve on what Mother Nature hath wrought. One such

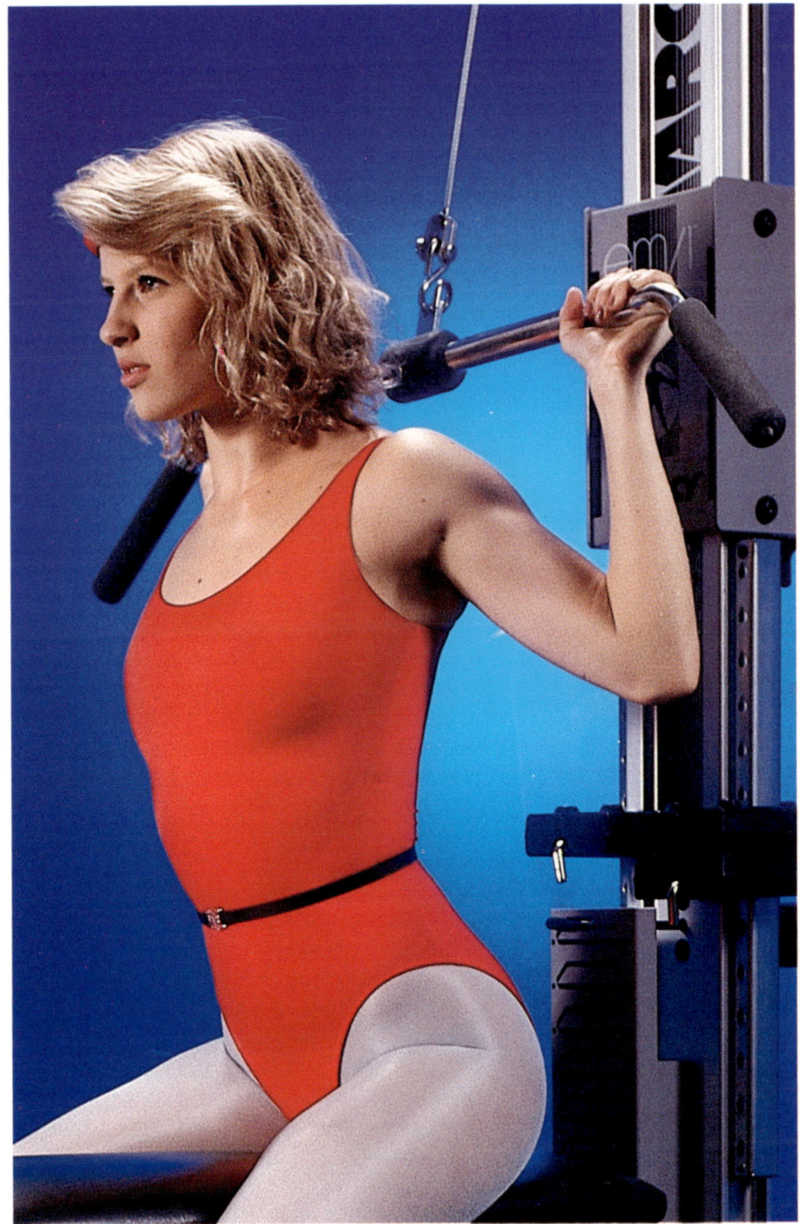

Pull-downs—a variation of chin-ups—allow you to vary the amount of weight hefted while developing upper back strength.

"improvement" on nature was developed before the turn of the century. It wasn't used extensively until recently, however, when Nautilus and other manufacturers began playing with offset cams that look like lopsided pulleys.

VARIABLE RESISTANCE DEVICES

When you hoist a weight by pulling on a cable that goes over the top of a pulley and is attached to a weight, you're engaged in *constant resistance training.* If the pulley isn't round, or if the hole in the pulley isn't in the center, the amount of weight you lift at different points in your movement will change because the lopsided pulley—the offset cam—changes the leverage for you. Clever scientists during the latter part of the 1800s found that they could vary the resistance this way and make the variance coincide with the natural variance in each joint's leverage. In other words, they were able to make the amount of weight increase or decrease to coincide with the increase or decrease in musculoskeletal leverage during an exercise movement. This is *variable resistance training.*

As with constant resistance training, however, variable resistance training has its advantages as well as disadvantages. One major disadvantage is that the movement is not natural, and therefore causes "confusion" in the brain centers that interpret the force and movement pattern. The result, according to some experts, is that muscular gains in strength and size are slower in coming and are limited in their final potential

Another major disadvantage—one shared by all exercise machines, regardless of their underlying technology—is that because the movement pattern is directed for you, surrounding muscles that act as *stabilizers* and *assistants* are not stressed and therefore never have the chance to grow. This is not the way Mother Nature intended things to be. In every natural body movement you use far more than one muscle, many of which are meant to help control the movement pattern or assist in moving the resistance. Others act as stabilizers of the trunk or limbs so that the main muscle(s) can act more efficiently. None of these other important muscles are provided with sufficient stress to force them to become bigger, stronger, or more enduring when using machines that do the balancing or controlling of the weight for you.

This disadvantage is the chief reason why some serious athletes and bodybuilders most frequently opt for free weights—dumbbells and barbells—in their training. Of course, there are several exercises that do not lend themselves to free weight training, and machines then become most desirable. In fact, a great majority of professional athletes and bodybuilders use a *combination* of machines and free weights in their training, but with emphasis primarily on free weights.

But let's get back to variable resistance technology. There are many forms of variable resistance for exercise equipment. Cams and elliptical pulleys are but two. Another that has become extremely popular is the Dynamic Variable Resistance technology developed by Universal.

Universal's DVR machinery operates on the same theory as Nautilus's and Paramount's offset cams, but uses instead a rolling lever system. As you lift a weight on Universal's machines, the lever arm becomes shorter or longer by action of a rolling fulcrum point. Like the offset cam, the rolling fulcrum allows you to match your musculoskeletal leverage changes to the variations in resistance afforded by the machine. This is the major advantage of all variable resistance devices.

To understand why varying the resistance through an exercise movement is advantageous, recall one of the most important basic principles of conditioning listed on page 100. Principle 6, the overload principle, states that you can maximize the level of stress you place on your muscles by making them work as hard as possible throughout the full range of motion in any given exercise. That is precisely what variable resistance machines do.

To demonstrate this important advantage, let's try the same exercise discussed earlier, the deep-knee bend, or *squat*. Lower your body to a squatting position and begin to raise back up to a standing position. Notice that near the bottom of the squat your leverage is poorest, and you can move less weight than near the top where your leverage is best. That means that your leg muscles are only benefiting near the bottom because the stress is greatest there. The stress on your leg muscles becomes less and less as you ascend back to a standing position. In fact, the stress becomes so minimal that virtually no gain in strength, size, or endurance is likely. Why? Because you have not stressed your muscles more than they are usually stressed (principle 1).

With variable resistance machines, the stress is increased throughout the ascent from the squat position and matches the improvement in your musculoskeletal leverage. The result is that you are now receiving ample overload stress to make your muscles work more than usual, so growth occurs.

Literally scores of other forms of variable resistance devices have found their way into the fitness marketplace. Springs, rubber bands, surgical tubing, and a host of other home-use and health-club-quality contraptions all make your job of picking the most suitable equipment more difficult.

SPRINGS:

Stretching a spring becomes more difficult the more it's stretched. As long as the increasing difficulty matches your improving leverage through an exercise movement, it will be effective as an exercise device. This rarely happens, though, and springs are therefore relegated to a position of lesser effectiveness as a form of resistance.

RUBBER BANDS AND SURGICAL TUBING:

The most popular form of stretch resistance is manufactured by Soloflex. Their machine uses elastic bands for its source of resistance. If you want more resistance, you simply add more elastic bands. Devices such as the Soloflex apparatus hand-held elastic stretch devices and the like are *in my opinion,* no more effective than the spring mentioned above, and their popularity is due more to their low cost and aggressive marketing than their effectiveness.

The biggest drawback of variable resistance devices, apart from their unnatural feel, is that it is quite impossible to perfectly match the variance in human muscoloskeletal leverage by manipulating the resistance you apply. People come in all shapes and sizes, and their leverage systems vary as much. This makes it quite impossible to match human leverage with machine leverage, making the concept of variable resistance theoretical at best. Rolling lever systems such as Universal's, and offset cams such as Paramount's, Nautilus's, and others come closest, however. Remember that all of these devices are effective—some more than others.

ACCOMMODATING RESISTANCE DEVICES

The fitness industry's war of one-upmanship rages on. The newest form of resistance to hit the marketplace is called *accommodating resistance.* Like variable resistance devices, accommodating resistance machinery is designed to allow you to exert maximum resistance throughout the full range of movement in each of your exercises. In so doing, you are able to maximize the amount of exercise stress your muscles receive. But there is a big difference: While variable resistance devices operate on the theory that the amount of resistance changes to match the leverage changes in your body, accommodating resistance maintains the resistance by *controlling the speed* of your exercise movement.

When you push on a weight that can go only at a fixed rate of speed, it doesn't matter what your leverage is—you will be able to exert maximum force in any position. Even though you can exert more force at the top of a squat movement than you can at the bottom, with accommodating resistance technology you will be able to maximize the amount of muscular force being applied throughout the entire squat movement.

Of course, the advantage gained in being able to apply maximum overload force throughout the entire range of each exercise movement is that you are now able to increase the amount of *time* that adaptive overload is applied in each exercise. But is that really an advantage?

Some exercise scientists say no, that the accommodating resistance technology is no more than another marketing gimmick to improve sales. But if you heed the arguments of their inventors—almost all of whom are like crusaders in their zeal—time is a critical element of overload, almost as important as *tension. Tension* (resistance that is stressful enough to cause muscles to adapt) together with sufficient *time* over which it is applied go hand in hand to produce superior gains, they say. A true statement to be sure, but it implies that the time over which overload is applied with other machines of the constant resistance and variable resistance varieties is inadequate. Such is not the case, and it's fair to say that all three technologies are very effective. Each has its distinct advantages and disadvantages.

The one feature that all accommodating resistance device manufacturers claim as the chief advantage of controlled speed exercise is the fact that it eliminates ballistic movement. (Ballistic movement is the thrust movement.) This, they say, improves the quality of overload throughout the exercise movement and eliminates, as well, the danger resulting from overextended joints, uncontrolled movements, or pulled muscles.

As with variable resistance devices, however, accommodating resistance movements are unnatural and therefore limited in their effectiveness. It seems that the brain isn't adapted to accepting the unnaturalness of controlled speed; ballistic movements are the way nature intended muscles and joints to work. Taking a look at how controlled speed training is accomplished provides a clue as to why some scientists believe this to be true.

The Cam II and Cam III machines manufactured by Kaiser use compressed air to control movement speed. The advantage of using air is that it can be moved very rapidly to and from a storage reservoir, making it possible to precisely control resistance at any point in an exercise movement, and rather quickly. As fatigue sets in, for example, reducing the amount of air pressure by routing some air back to the storage reservoir makes it possible to continue exercising. This can be accomplished by the press of a button or pedal conveniently located on the machine.

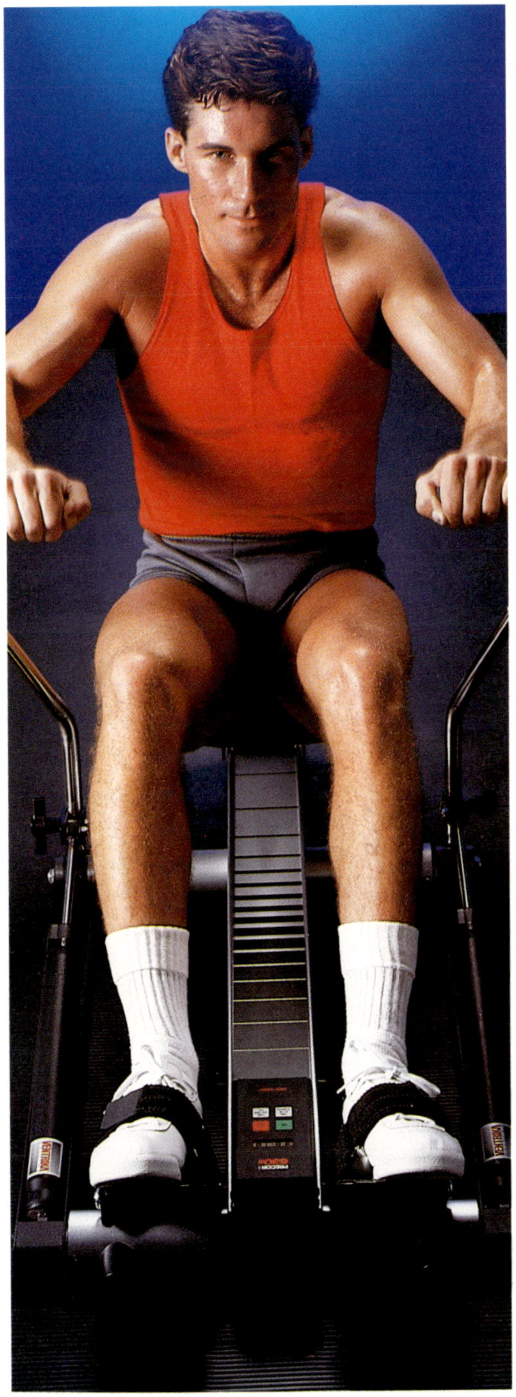

Rowing machines used to be a common fixture in gyms everywhere. They're making a comeback. Why? Because it's great full-body exercise!

Several different machines use friction to control speed. The Mini-Gym uses a combination of clutch plates and flywheel, and speed can be controlled by reducing or increasing the amount of friction between the clutch plates. Unlike the Kaiser equipment, you have to stop exercising to adjust the tension (speed). Exercise bicycles use friction as well. The Stairwalker, a relative newcomer to the world of exercise technology, also employs friction. This ingenious device allows you to walk upstairs—quickly or slowly—without having to return to the bottom for another set! It resembles a miniature escalator. The Bullworker became famous as the exercise device used aboard the Apollo spacecraft. It too uses friction as its source of resistance. A rope wound around a central rod is pulled during exercise. The more winds of the rope, the more friction. Though electric treadmills of the sort used in scientific laboratories control speed by electric motors, manual treadmills use friction to control walking or running speed.

Yet another accommodating resistance apparatus uses fluid cylinders similar to a car's shock absorbers. By adjusting the hole diameter through which the fluid passes you can vary the speed of movement. The most noteworthy example of this sort of technology is found in the Hydra-Gym line. Their equipment can, like Kaiser's, be adjusted without interrupting your exercise. Practically all rowing machines on the market use fluid in the same way the Hydra-Gym does.

The plethora of devices finding their way into today's fitness marketplace are testimony to the incredible popularity the fitness craze enjoys today. It's safe to say that nearly all of these devices work. They all can, if used *properly* and *consistently,* help you to attain a level of fitness greater than that with which you started. Most offer miraculous results, but in the final analysis it's *you* who must do the work! *No machine yet developed can do that for you.*

STATIC RESISTANCE DEVICES

Contracting your muscles without movement is called *static contraction.* The term *isometric exercise* was coined to describe this form of stress. During the fifties and early sixties, this form of exercise was heralded as a major technological breakthrough. In bandwagon fashion, athletes the world over—even the suspicious Soviets—adopted isometric exercise as a major strength-building technique. The public obligingly followed their lead.

It wasn't too long before the truth was learned. Isometrically contracting a muscle—pushing or pulling on immovable apparatus—made you strong *only in that position*! In order to become stronger throughout the entire range of movement, you would have to pull or push at every angle throughout the entire range! Of course, this was impossible from a practical as well as technological standpoint. The isometric movement died a quiet death.

It seems that the nerves running from the brain and spinal column to the muscles are not capable of delivering an electrochemical impulse in ranges of movement other than that for which they are made. To make a muscle bigger, stronger, or more enduring, the exercise scientists found you must stress the muscle through the entire range of movement.

Still, static muscle contraction does make you stronger in the position to which it's applied, and therefore has some uses in sports training. Because of the extreme stress such training has on the heart—blood flow is all but stopped in the statically contracting muscle—isometric exercise is not recommended for those with heart problems or high blood pressure.

Some Noteworthy Devices

There are many fitness devices on the market that are designed to deliver cardiovascular benefits, chiropractic (spinal) fitness, and sports skill. Often, these devices are difficult to categorize on the basis of the four technologies of fitness equipment discussed earlier. Let's review some of them, as you will surely run into many of them in your quest for fitness.

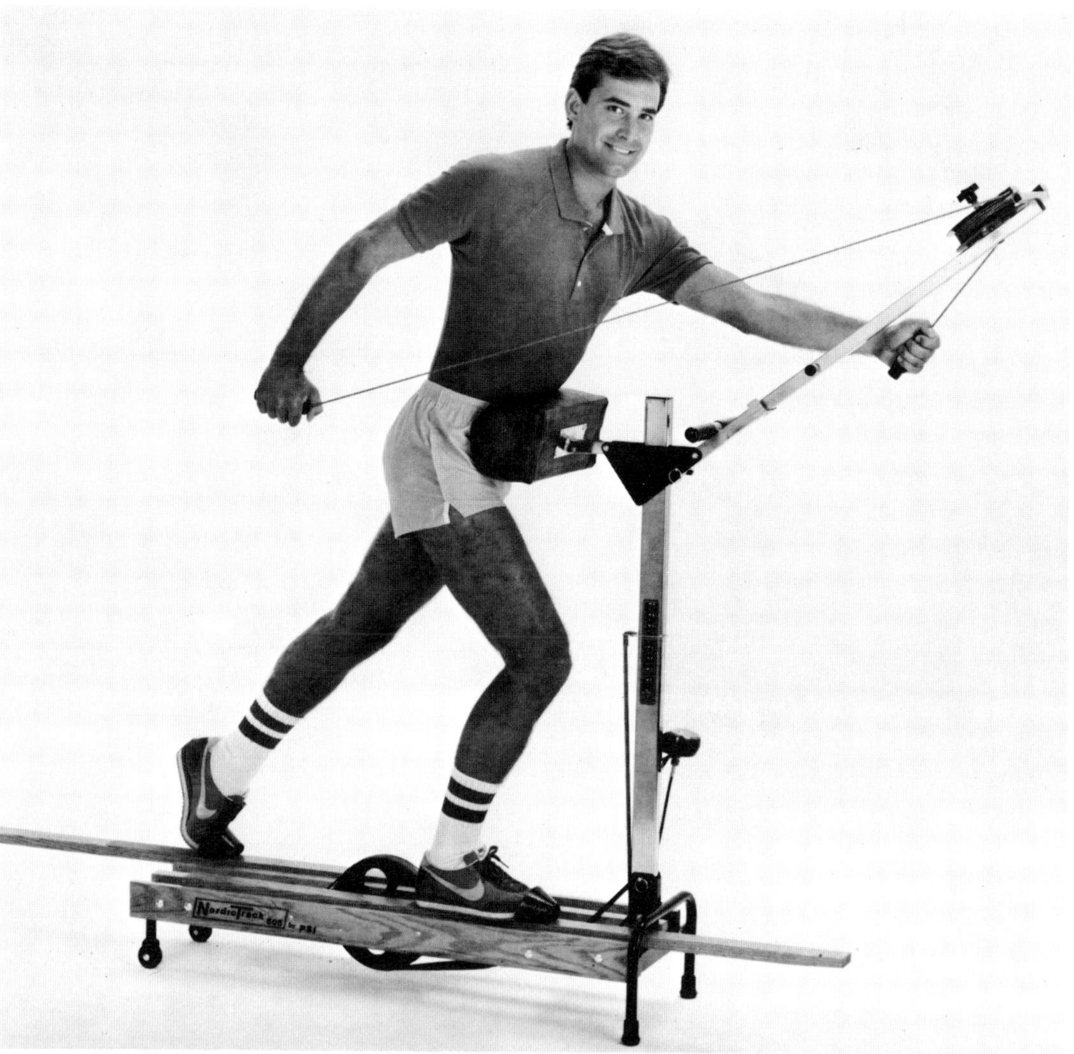

Any time you use your own body weight as a source of resistance, you are using constant resistance technology. Push-ups, pull-ups, jumping jacks, even stretching, fall into this category. Sometimes special apparatuses facilitate calisthenic exercise. The *dancer's barre*, *chin-up bars*, *twisting platforms*, *hand springs*, *slant boards* for sit-ups, *skipping ropes*, *inversion machines*, and *miniature trampolines* are but a few of the well-known calisthenic apparatuses on the market today.

Some calisthenic exercises are designed to improve endurance (either cardiovascular or in a single muscle group), strength, or flexibility. Others, like the NordicTrack ski simulator and the *roller ski shoes*, are designed to deliver both cardiovascular benefits as well as sports skill. Another example of sports skill calisthenics is the agility drill. Even running and jogging are considered calisthenic exercise because you use your own body weight. Adding *Heavyhands or ankle weights* makes running more stressful.

If there are no springs, offset cams, shock absorbers, or other devices attached to vary or control movement, then calisthenic exercises are actually a special application of constant resistance technology. The reason is quite simple: If your body weight is sufficiently heavy, it delivers overload to the muscles. In this light, then, calisthenics are just like constant resistance weight training.

The most important point to remember about calisthenics is that if your muscles do not receive more stress than what they are used to, you are wasting your time. *You will not benefit from non-stressful exercise.* If a calisthenic movement is too easy, simply begin using free weights or machines. Weight training takes up where calisthenics leave off.

The remainder of this chapter focuses on actual training exercises. Each exercise is discussed fully, both with regard to what muscle(s) is affected and which machines work best. Remember that all of the technologies employed in weight training have advantages and disadvantages. You must select exercises and apparatuses that help you achieve the maximum benefit. The chart (right) will give you this author's opinions on the relative usefulness of different kinds of exercise equipment in achieving your training goals.

TRAINING OBJECTIVE EFFECTIVENESS RATINGS

BODYBUILDING EQUIPMENT EFFECTIVENESS

There is no question that machines are an integral part of the fitness scene, but for maximum bodybuilding benefits, how do the different equipment types stack up? The author has applied his own ratings to each kind of device as it serves the basic objectives of weight training in your lifestyle.

(on a scale of 1–10)	DUMBBELLS & BARBELLS	CONSTANT RESISTANCE MACHINES	CLUTCH & FLYWHEEL MACHINES	AIR & HYDRAULIC MACHINES	CAM MACHINES	LEVER MACHINES
Muscular size increases	10	8	7	9	4	4
Muscular strength increases	10	7	6	8	6	6
Explosive power increases	8	5	5	5	9	9
Sport skills carryover for the movement employed	9	5	5	5	5	7
Sport skills carryover for the velocity/acceleration employed	9	5	3	5	4	4
Quality of overload through the entire exercise set	6	6	7	7	8	8
Quality of muscular isolation	10	8	8	8	8	8
Overall versatility	10	6	5	6	5	6
TOTAL EFFECTIVENESS SCORE	72	50	46	53	49	52
	constant resistance		variable resistance		accommodating resistance	

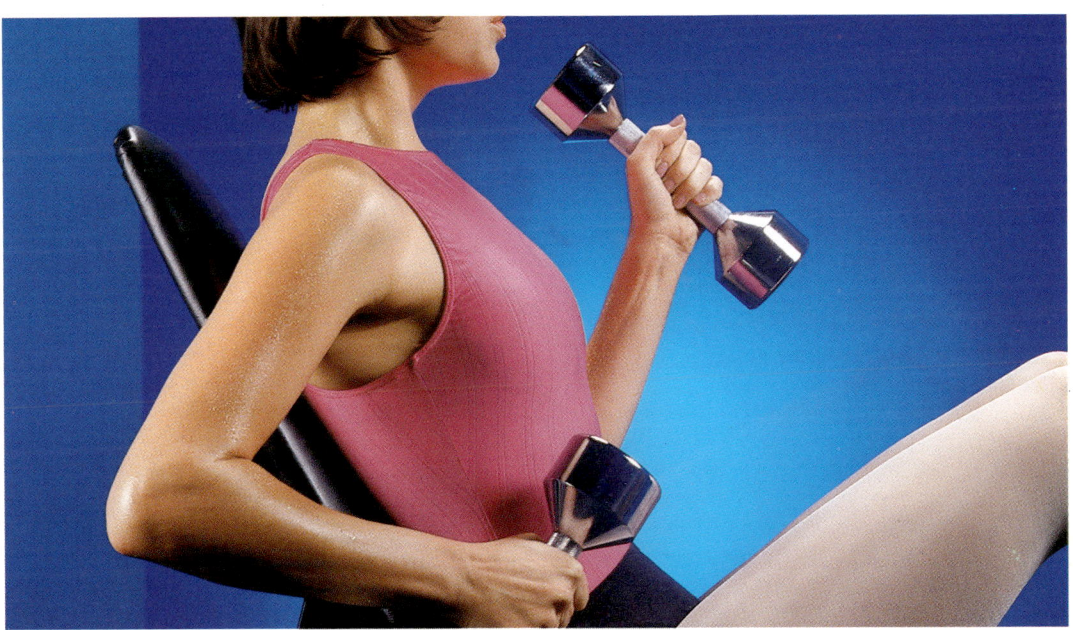

Dumbbells remain the choice equipment among weight-training aficionados for upper body workouts. They're cheap, portable, and can be used on several types of benches.

The Major Exercises for Each Part of Your Body

This section focuses on the actual exercises: those which are best for each body part and which muscles are affected. Remember, practically *any* exercise is better than none. Some types of exercise equipment work better than others, just as some exercise movements work better than others. Try to keep the basic principles of conditioning in mind when reading the following exercise descriptions, and it will become clear to you why some movements work better than others.

The exercises here relate to the major segments (muscles) of the body:

- chest
- shoulders
- upper arms
- forearms
- upper back
- lower back
- sides
- abdominals
- hips
- thighs
- lower legs

Since there are several muscles involved in each of these major body segments, there are often several exercises that can be appropriate. However, those discussed here are the most important ones, and any complete fitness or sports conditioning program will include them. Others are included frequently, but not until advanced fitness or conditioning is achieved.

COMPARISON BETWEEN MACHINES AND FREE WEIGHTS

Advantages of Free Weights

- Dumbbells and barbells are more effective in developing the smaller synergistic (helping) muscles and stabilizer muscles.
- Free weight exercises more closely match the neurological patterns of associated sports skills because of joint kinesthesis, leverage similarities, and bodily involvement, from a biomechanical point of view.
- Barbells and dumbbells are more versatile.
- Barbells and dumbbells are less expensive.
- Barbells and dumbbells take up less space (for home gym use).
- Greater overall strength can be achieved using barbells and dumbbells.
- Power is improved more efficiently and to a greater extent through the use of free weights.
- Other aspects of fitness, including size, flexibility, reduced body fat, and muscle toning are achieved more efficiently through the use of free weights.

Disadvantages of Barbell and Dumbbell Training

- Training alone can be dangerous; the heavy weights can cause injury if control is lost.
- Barbells and dumbbells that are adjustable can come apart if care is not taken to tightly secure the collars.
- Adjustments in weight from set to set requires affixing or removing plates and replacing and removing collars—often a time-consuming and tedious ordeal.
- You need large spaces to use barbells and dumbbells; it can be hazardous for large groups of unorganized people to use them in a small area.
- In certain exercises, it is difficult, if not impossible, to derive maximum isolation of a muscle or muscle group.

Advantages of Machines

- Some machines are more efficient in maximally isolating a muscle or muscle group for more efficient overload.
- Machines are generally safer than free weights because the weights are controlled by slides and held in place by retaining pins.
- For group use, some machines are more efficient in terms of space utilization (especially Universal machines).
- Machines are easier to use, and therefore faster workouts are possible. Less time is usually wasted changing plates and waiting for spotters. For the average fitness enthusiast seeking reasonable tonus and strength, machines generally prove to be more efficient; it's easier to get in a "lunch hour" workout on a machine.

Disadvantages of Machines

- All machines are not alike in every regard, but most require the moving of a weight along a predetermined path (or track), making it nearly impossible to derive synergistic or stabilizer muscle strength.
- Machines that control movement velocity (such as isokinetic machines) or vary the resistance over a given movement (such as Nautilus or Universal machines), have removed the "natural" aspect from the exercise, which many physiologists claim renders such machines less effective in developing strength and size—differing neurological input is the chief reason cited.
- Because of machine construction constraints, it is generally impossible to achieve maximum velocity—and high-speed training is often a prerequisite in sports training. The machines would either break, jerk about violently, or simply not accommodate such training.
- Most machines are constructed to serve the average-sized person—very short or very tall people find it almost impossible to use many of the machines currently on the market, particularly Nautilus machines.
- Machines tend to be in a price range beyond the means of many gym owners, and often beyond the means of commercial spas as well.
- Many machines are so specialized that one would have to purchase several in order to get even a marginally effective workout—floor space and budget permitting.
- Space-age appearance of many machines lull users into believing that high technology equals maximum efficiency in achieving fitness goals—a sentiment that is definitely not true. Nothing beats hard work.

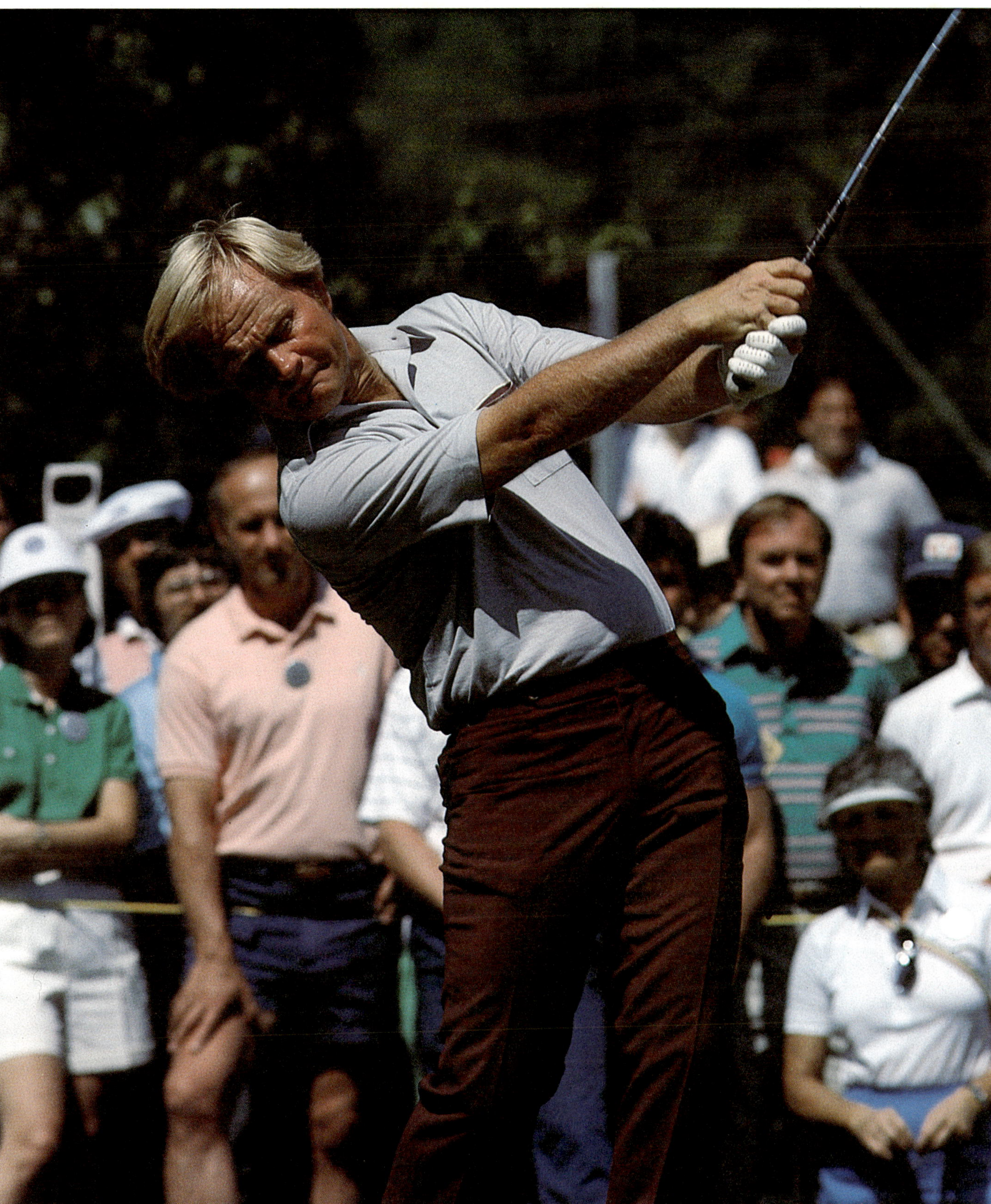

Golfer Jack Nicklaus needs a powerful form, so regularly works out to maintain his strength and endurance.

BODY PART

CHEST

TARGET MUSCLES:
Clavicular pectoralis (upper chest)
Sternal pectoralis (lower chest)

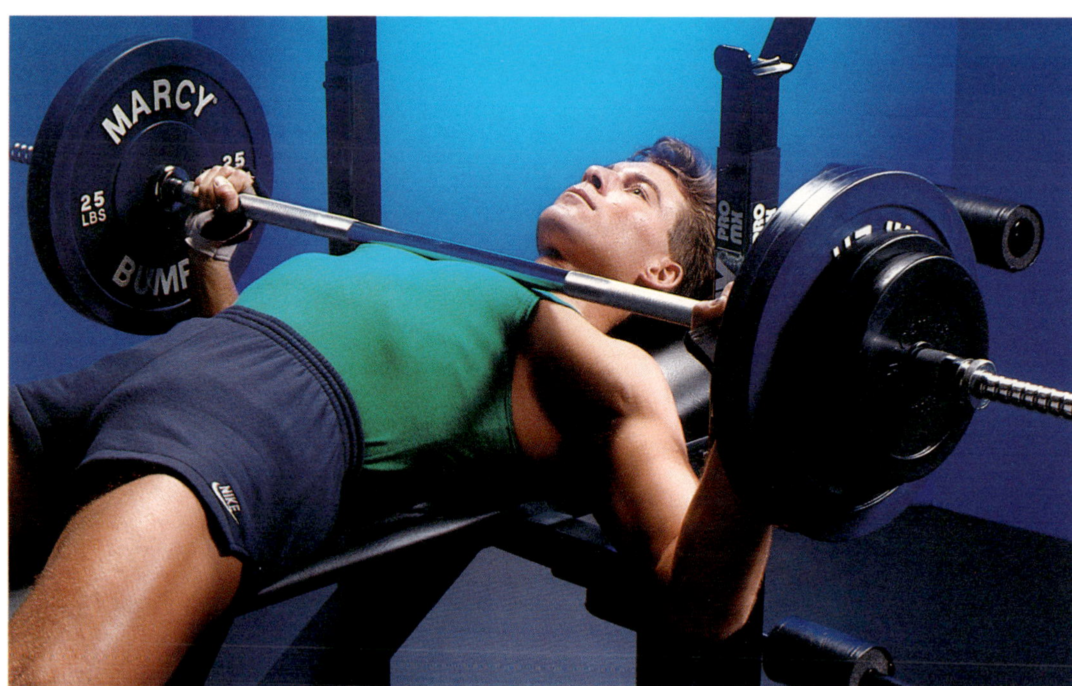

Free Weight Exercises:
Bench presses with dumbbells or barbells are performed while lying on a bench (supine position). These exercises are considered the best way to develop both the upper and lower chest. One drawback is that the triceps (back of upper arm) and front deltoid (front shoulder) muscles are also affected, and can sometimes limit bench press efforts. A great way to get maximum isolation of the chest muscles is to do *flyes* with dumbbells. The major advantage of bench presses and flyes is that surrounding muscles, which help balance and control the weight, are also developed, an important consideration for athletes. Bench presses *must* be performed with a spotter (a partner) standing ready to assist in case you fail to make the lift. The exercise can be extremely dangerous!

Machine Exercises:
Bench presses can be performed on Universal's DVR machine, Paramount, Soloflex, Marcy, or DP equipment. All are similar to regular bench presses done with the free weights, except that the path of the exercise movement is controlled; remember, "helped" muscles receive little or no benefit. There are some equipment manufacturers, (like Nautilus, Kaiser, and Universal), who make a machine called the *pec Deck,* which allows isolation of the pectoralis muscles while in a seated (rather than supine) position. All are quite effective, but free weight exercises are generally regarded as the most effective way to develop the chest.

BODY PART

SHOULDERS

TARGET MUSCLES:
Deltoids
(front, middle, and rear shoulders)

Free Weight Exercises:
Lateral raises with dumbbells (raise the two dumbbells sideward to head height) and *upright rows* with a barbell (with hands close together, lift the barbell to your chin) are two favorite shoulder exercises among bodybuilders and athletes. To center more on the front shoulder muscles, raise the dumbbells or barbell frontward to head height. To affect the rear deltoids, *inverted flyes* (with dumbbells in hand, bend forward and raise the dumbbells sideward) are recommended. Again, experts feel that free weight exercises are the most efficient because they exercise many muscles at the same time.

Machine Exercises:
Several companies, including Universal, Nautilus, Marcy, DP, Paramount, and others, have seated or standing *military press* stations on their equipment. This exercise does affect the shoulders (primarily the middle deltoid), but you will almost always be limited in your efforts by the weaker tricep muscles (in the back of the upper arm). Nautilus, Kaiser, and a few others feature a seated deltoid raise machine (middle deltoid) that works quite well in achieving maximum isolation of the target muscles. Almost all of the major equipment manufacturers have a low pulley attachment that allows you to do upright rows or one-side-at-a-time lateral raises with a cable system—these exercises are also quite effective. No single machine stands out as better than the rest when it comes to effectively exercising the shoulder muscles.

BODY PART

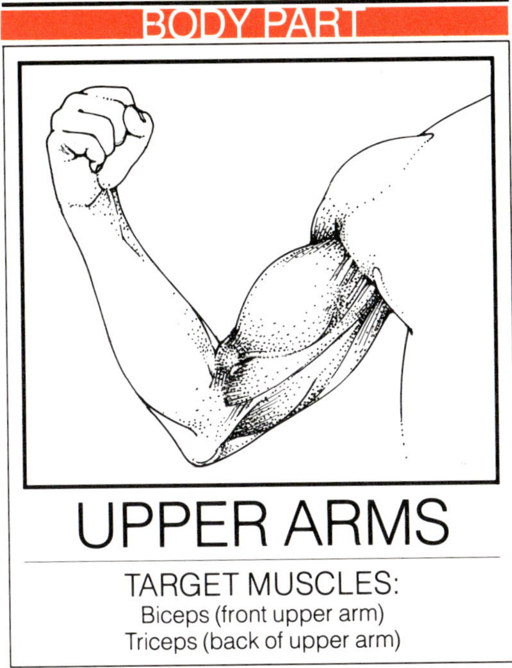

UPPER ARMS

TARGET MUSCLES:
Biceps (front upper arm)
Triceps (back of upper arm)

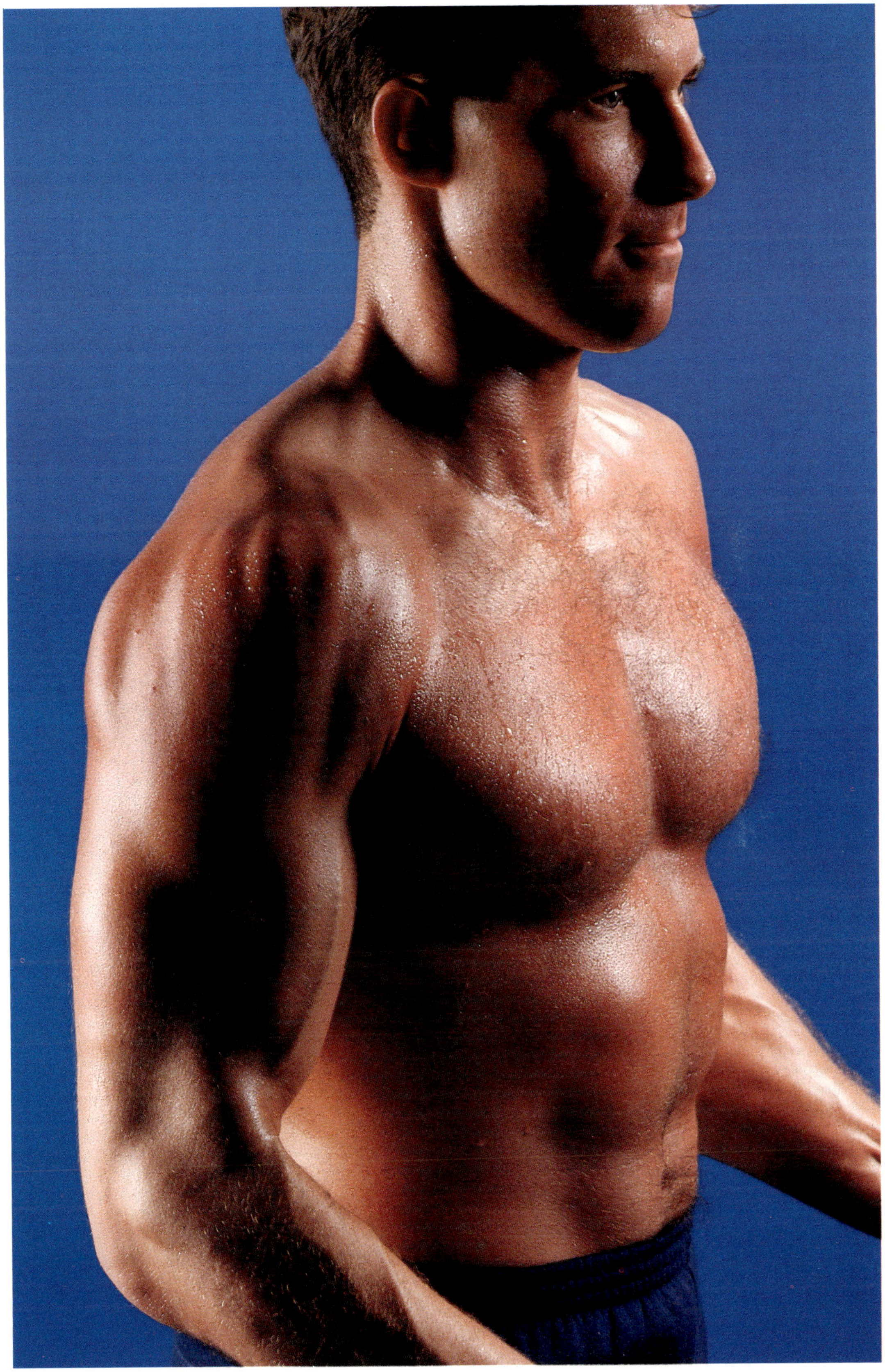

Free Weight Exercises:

Bicep curls (bend the elbows with dumbbells or a barbell in hand) and *tricep extensions* (while lying on your back, straighten the arms to an overhead position) are the most effective exercises for the muscles of the upper arms. Many muscles in the shoulder girdle help and control during the execution of these two popular exercises, making them exceptionally suited for athletes and bodybuilders. Several variations of these two basic movements have become popular; some can be performed with machines.

Machine Exercises:

Nautilus, Paramount, Marcy, and Kaiser (to name a few) have developed *Scott curl machines* (also called *preacher curl machines*) for the biceps. Several, including those mentioned, have adapted the machines to accommodate *tricep pushdowns.* The common name for these machines is the *double arm machine.* All are quite effective, but they share the disadvantage of not being adjustable enough to fit very short and very tall users. As with all machines, variable resistance, accommodating resistance, and constant resistance technology is employed. Your choice of which is most suited to your needs depends on your training goals, and, more important, on personal preference.

BODY PART

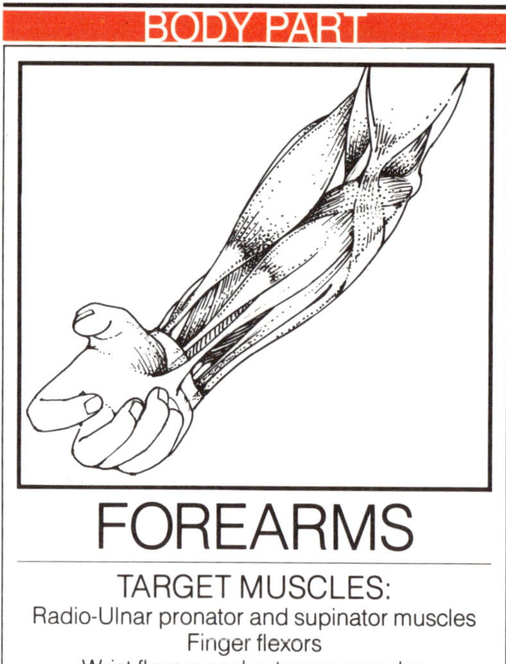

FOREARMS

TARGET MUSCLES:
Radio-Ulnar pronator and supinator muscles
Finger flexors
Wrist flexors and extensor muscles

Free Weight Exercises:

For wrist flexors, rest the forearms on a bench with palms facing upward, and raise the barbell upward by flexing the wrist. For wrist extensors, rest the forearms on a bench with palms facing downward, and raise the barbell by extending the wrists. Even with very light weights, your forearms will feel a deep burning sensation, a signal of development taking place. The same sensation is experienced with forearm pronations (forearms rotating to a palms-up position), both of which use a dumbbell handle with weights on one end only, called a *Thor's Hammer.*

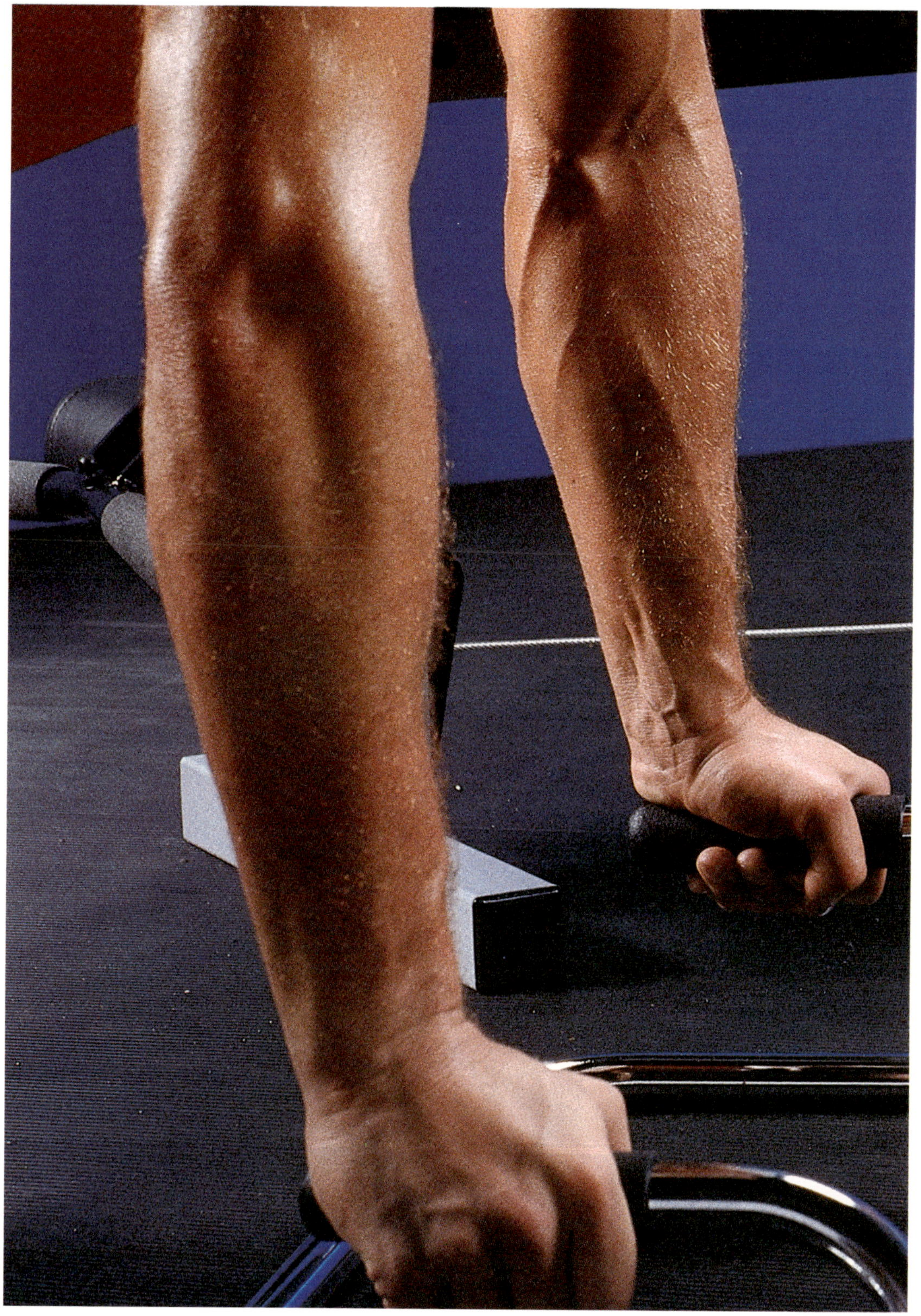

Machine Exercises:

The only machines for the forearms presently on the market are called *wrist rollers.* Made by Marcy, Paramount, and others, this device is a simple rope tied to weights at its bottom and a roller at the top. The object is to roll the rope around the roller, which in turn raises the weight. It's effective, but, in my opinion, cumbersome and expensive; free weights are more versatile. This device only develops the wrist extensor muscles—flexors, pronators, and supinators are left unaffected. There are many *gripping* devices on the market that develop the finger flexors (which are located in the forearms). These include springs, rubber balls, and various other squeezable devices that employ constant resistance technology. All are very good, and there seems to be no discernible advantage in any particular type. The free weight exercises are best, primarily because of their versatility.

BODY PART

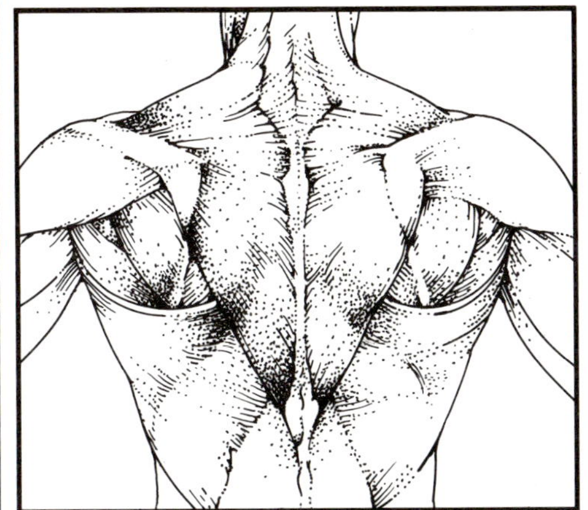

UPPER BACK

TARGET MUSCLES:
Latissimus dorsi
(arm depressor muscles)
Rhomboids
(downward rotators of the scapulae)
Trapezius (shoulder elevators)

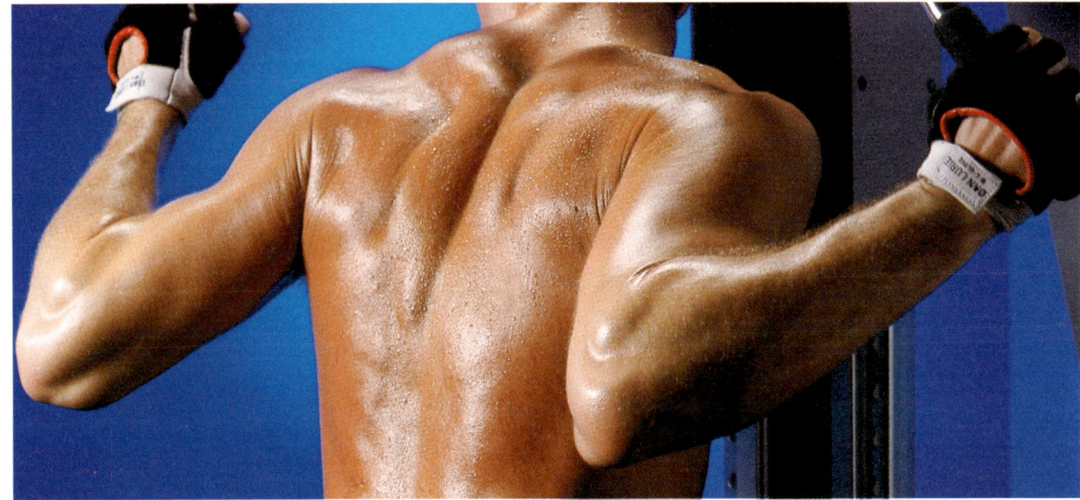

Free Weight Exercises:

Chin-ups, a calisthenic movement, are the most popular exercise for the latissimus dorsi muscles (called *lats* for short). Of course, you must be able to lift your own body weight to do them! *Bent rows* are done for the rhomboids (bend forward and pull a barbell to your chest so that the elbows are at a 90-degree angle from your body). Your ability to perform this movement is often limited if your biceps are weaker than your rhomboids, however, but *inverted flyes* (bend forward and raise two dumbbells to the side) can be performed when bicep weakness limits your ability to do bent rows. To develop the trapezius muscles, hold a barbell in front of you and rest it against your thighs while shrugging the shoulders upward (these are called *shrugs*). If you feel a burning sensation brought on by fatigue on top of your shoulders close to the neck, you know you're doing it right.

Machine Exercises:

Lat pull-downs are performed by pulling down on a bar attached to an overhead cable. The cable is attached to weight stacks on most machines. Universal, Marcy, Paramount, and several other manufacturers make such a device and all employ constant resistance. When your body prohibits you from performing pull-ups, lat pull-downs are the best way to develop the lats. Also, when you are so strong that your body weight isn't sufficient for maximum stress, lat pull-downs again are the answer. Nautilus and a few other manufacturers make a *pull-over machine,* which is also effective in exercising the lats.

Nautilus, Marcy, Paramount, and others make a shrug machine, which requires you to rest your forearms in a padded lever device which, when the shrug movement is executed, raises a weight stack. I find this device almost always hurts my forearms where the pads rest on them, and in my opinion, is not a very appealing alternative to the more comfortable and effective barbell shrug exercise.

BODY PART

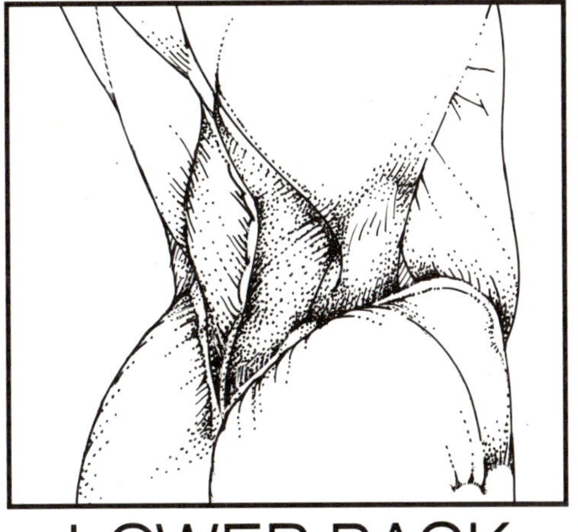

LOWER BACK

TARGET MUSCLES:
Erector spinae (two long muscles located on each side of your spine)

Free Weight Exercises:

Back extension and *deadlifts* are the two most popular lower-back exercises. To execute back extensions, hang face down over a waist-high bench with feet secured under a padded bar. Simply bend at the waist and then raise up with a small weight held behind the head to develop effectively the erector spinae muscles. Deadlifts (bend down and pick up a barbell to the erect position) also effectively develops the lower back. Care must be used in the latter exercise, so that too much stress is not placed on the relatively fragile spine. Slipping a disc can be a career-ending injury!

Machine Exercises:

Very few equipment manufacturers make lower-back machines. Can the reason be that lower-back problems are so prevalent that law suits would become a problem? There are a couple of notable exceptions, however. One is the Nautilus *low back machine* which, incidentally, is quite safe. A padded lever against your back raises a weight stack when you extend your body backward. As with all Nautilus's equipment, it uses variable resistance technology. It's a great device for general toning or lower-back endurance, but not nearly as suited to developing strength, size, or power as the free weight exercise.

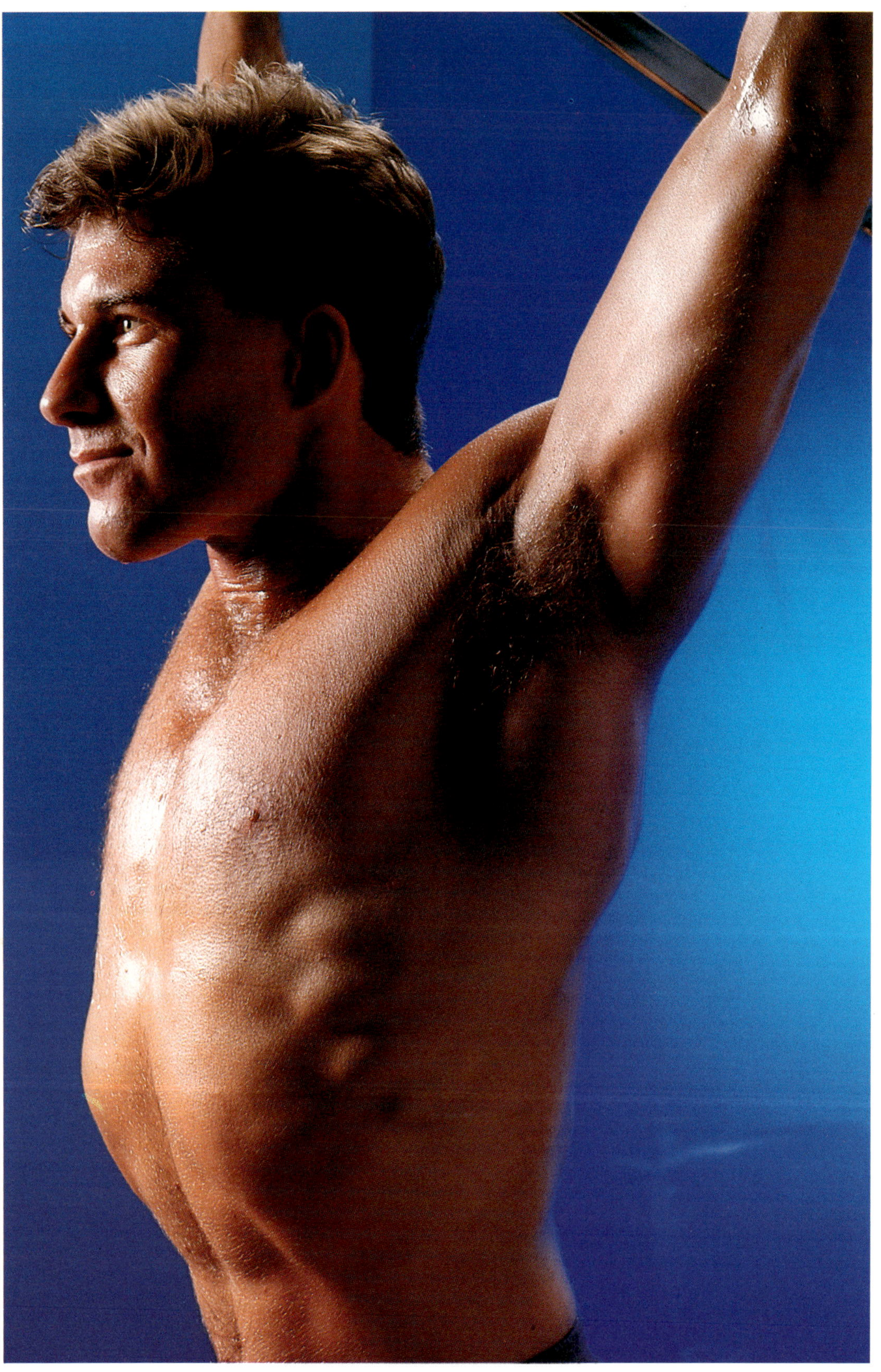

BODY PART

SIDES

TARGET MUSCLES:
Internal and external obliques (sides)
Quadratus lumborum
(lateral flexor of spine)

Free Weight Exercises:
Side bends are by far the most effective exercise for the muscles of the side, including the deeply located quadratus lumborum, an extremely important muscle for improving the stability of the lumbar vertebrae. Holding a dumbbell in one hand, bend to the weighted side, and then raise back to an erect position. This movement will develop the internal and external obliques on the unweighted side. Then perform the same movement with the weight held on the opposite side.

Machine Exercises:
Holding the handle of a cable attached to a low pulley works identically with the free weight side bends described above. Many equipment companies, including Marcy, Paramount, and DP, make a *twisting platform* that is designed to tone the muscles of the sides. Holding onto a set of handles or a Dancer's Barre in front of you while standing on the circular platform, simply twist from side to side, relying on your stopping and starting body inertia to provide overload stress to the internal and external obliques. But—unfortunately—the stress is too little to do any real good, and most important, the lumbar vertebrae take a severe beating with this side-to-side twisting. In this writer's opinion, it is a dangerous exercise and ought to be out-

lawed! In fairness, however, it should also be pointed out that twisting can *benefit* the muscles near the spine. Simply do them slowly with resistance provided by surgical tubing.

BODY PART

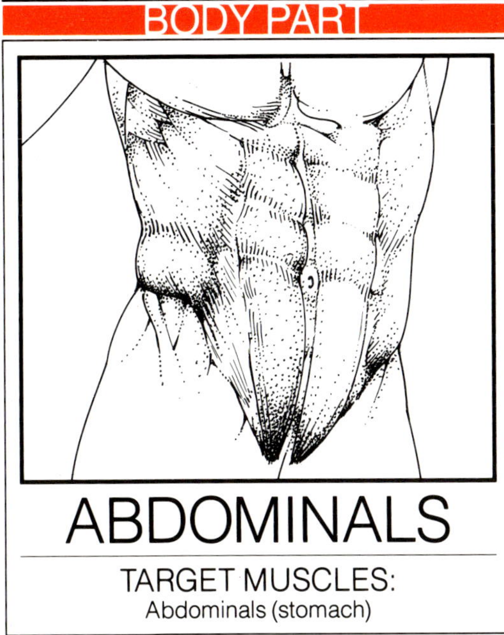

ABDOMINALS

TARGET MUSCLES:
Abdominals (stomach)

Free Weight Exercises:

Everyone knows what *sit-ups* are, but did you know that they are dangerous? Most people perform sit-ups in the hope that their bellies will flatten. In the process, they all but ruin their lumbar spine by action of a very strong hip flexor muscle called the *iliopsoas*. This muscle is the primary muscle involved in sitting-up movement—not the abdominals! All the abdominals do is stabilize the trunk by statically contracting. The best calisthenic exercise for the abdominals is the *crunch,* a partial sit-up performed with the hips already fully flexed. Lie on your back with your feet over the top of a bench and "crunch" your torso by drawing your ribs toward your pelvis with the abdominal muscles. You can hold a weight behind your head for added stress. It's a very effective exercise.

Machine Exercises:

After Fitness Systems Equipment Company came out with its *abdominal crunch machine,* several others followed suit. Nautilus's abdominal machine requires you to raise your knees and pull down with your shoulders against two resistance sources. In my opinion, it's an inferior design because it stresses the iliopsoas (and therefore the lumbar spine) too much. Universal has a similar device, one which eliminates the lumbar spine problems of Nautilus, but the range of movement is limited. Fitness System's machine is by far the best on the market; it's now being manufactured by Weider Health & Fitness, Inc. It features a full range of motion for the abdominal muscles without placing stress on the spine or shoulder girdle—the abdominals are completely isolated. This is one area where machines have a decided advantage over free weights or calisthenics.

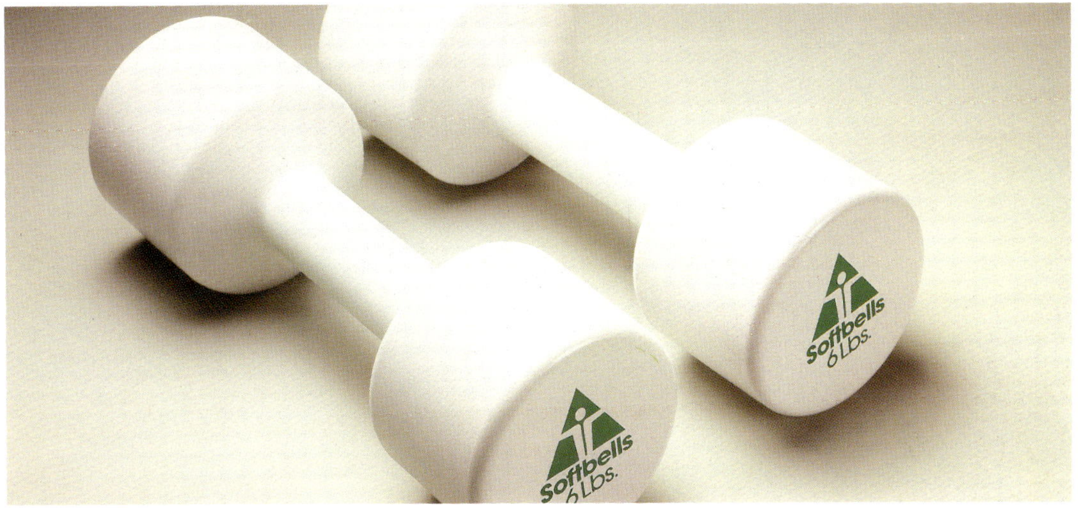

BODY PART

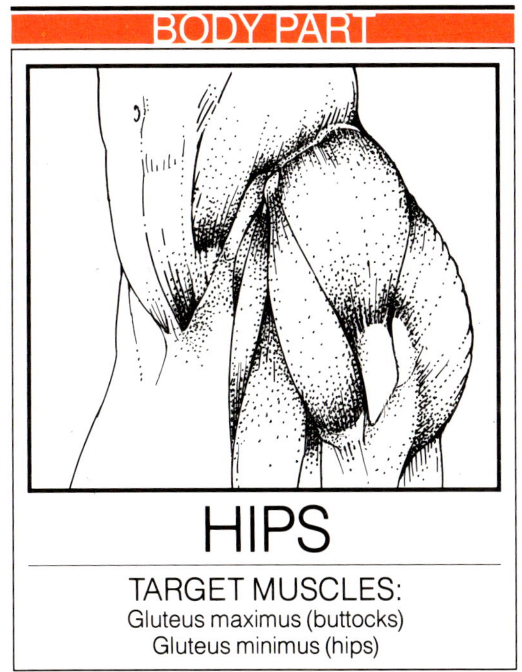

HIPS

TARGET MUSCLES:
Gluteus maximus (buttocks)
Gluteus minimus (hips)

Free Weight Exercises:

Stiff-legged deadlifts and *squats* effectively develop the gluteal muscles. In the process, the hamstrings and quadriceps of the upper legs and the erector spinae of the lower back are also exercised very effectively. Despite the fact that in these two exercise movements the gluteal muscles are not completely isolated, they are nonetheless very effective in strengthening and toning the target muscles. In fact, no other exercises, neither those employing free weights nor machines, are as effective as are squats and stiff-legged deadlifts. Partial squats never touch the gluteal muscles, and neither does the Stairmaster, despite the advertisements. Why? Because the hips have to be flexed almost all the way before the gluteals ever become stretched enough to afford a moving force! Climbing stairs (or using the Stairmaster) works the thigh muscles only. But, climbing stairs three at a time and with weights on your back would effectively develop gluteals.

Machine Exercises:

Several companies have developed reasonably effective gluteal machines. Nautilus's *hip and back machine,* like those made by Marcy and a few others, work to the extent they can tone the gluteal muscles. But none compare to squats and deadlifts, which develop strength, power, and endurance. The gluteus minimus can be effectively isolated and developed quite well with the *in-and-out thigh machine* made by Marcy and Paramount. The outward movement (hip abduction with outward rotation) targets the gluteus minimus.

BODY PART

THIGHS

TARGET MUSCLES:
Quadriceps (front of thighs)
Hamstrings (back of thighs)
Adductors (inside of thighs)
Abductors (outside of thighs up near the hips)

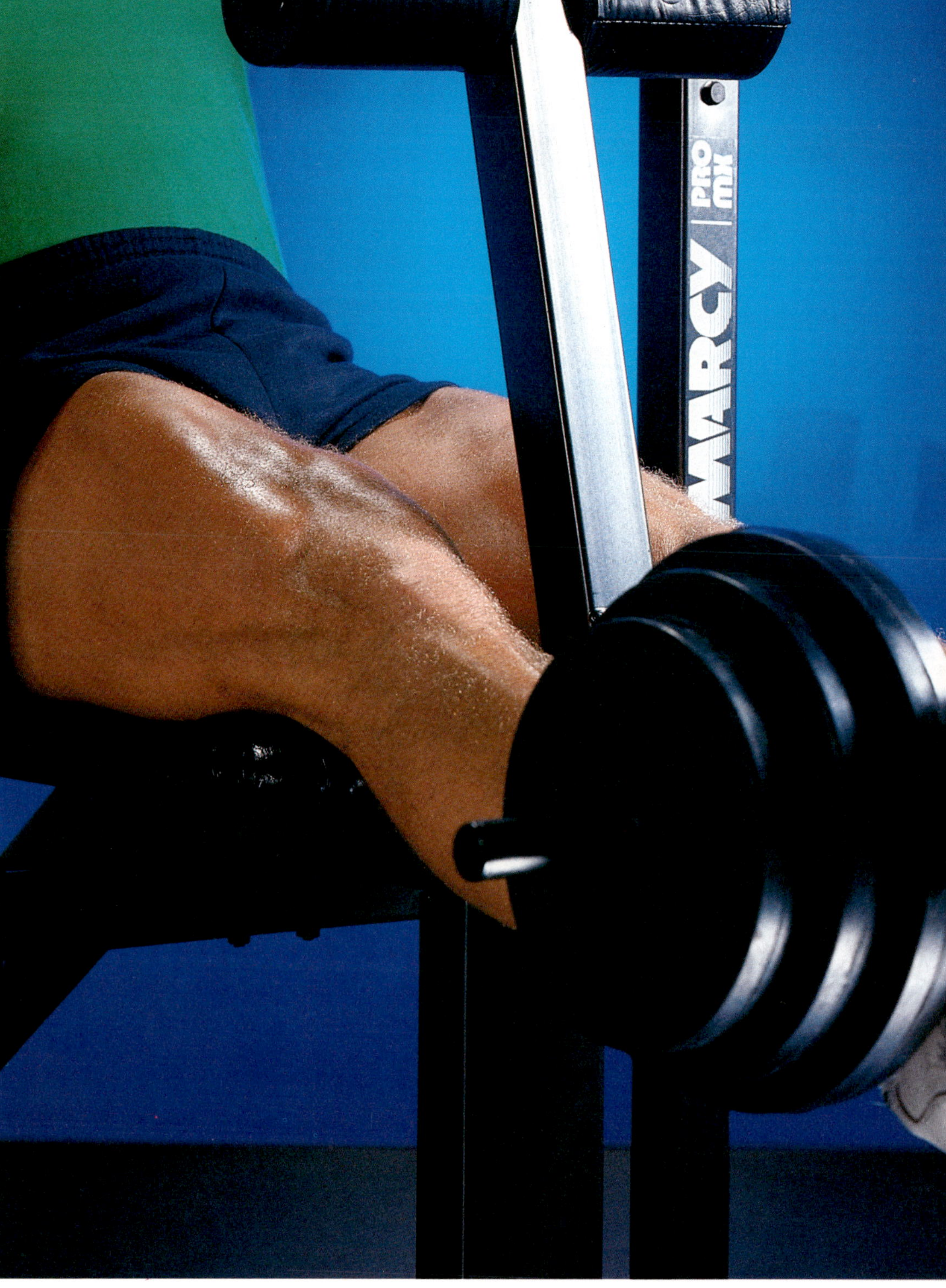

Free Weight Exercises:

As noted in the discussion on exercises for the hips, *squats* are excellent for the gluteals, hamstrings, and quadriceps. The adductor and abductor muscles of the inner and outer thighs are also exercised strongly in squats, as they provide assistance and stability during the movement. When done correctly, squats are by far the best exercise for all of the muscles of the thighs. No machine even comes close.

Machine Exercises:

Almost all of the major equipment companies manufacture *leg curl* and *leg extension benches* that attach to a weight stack and are operated with any one of the three technologies of weight training. These machines effectively isolate the hamstrings and quadriceps, respectively. In fact, they isolate them so well that very little weight can be lifted in these movements, making these exercises suitable only for toning, size, and endurance—not strength. If you want strength, you must do squats. Leg press machines, which require you to lie on your back and push a weight up or sit and push a weight up via lever action, are effective thigh developers. Nautilus, Universal, Marcy, Paramount, and a host of other manufacturers make such leg press machines. The in-and-out thigh machines manufactured by Marcy and Paramount are good for the gluteus minimus (hips) and the adductor muscles located on the inside of your thighs. Low pulley arrangements, on practi-

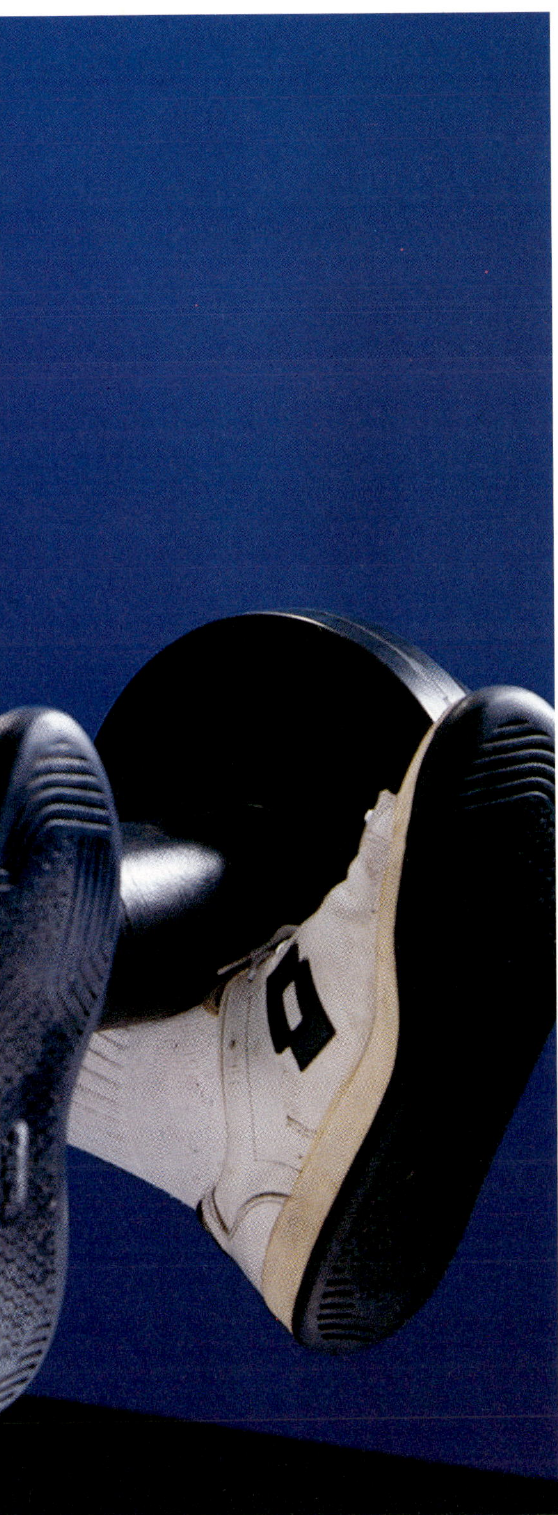

cally all commercial gym machines, are effectively used for the adductors and abductors (inside and outside of the thighs). An ankle strap allows leg kicks in all directions.

BODY PART

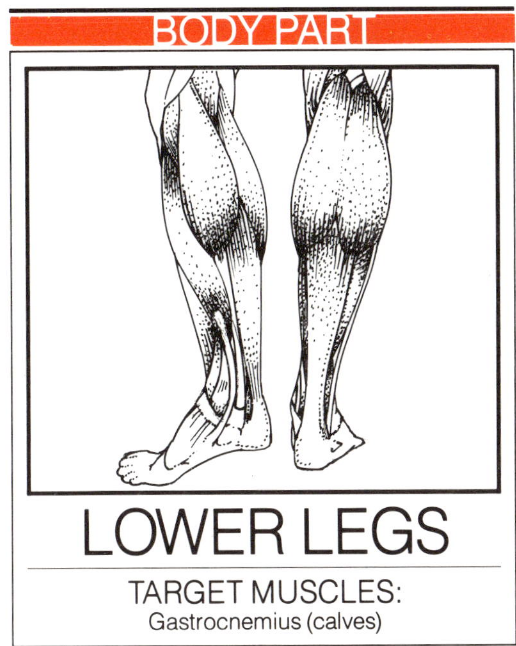

LOWER LEGS

TARGET MUSCLES:
Gastrocnemius (calves)

Free Weight Exercises:

Performing *toe raises* with a weight on your back develops the calves. But because your calves are very strong (owing to their great leverage), it is difficult to hold enough weight on your back to provide sufficient stress to force them to develop. The obvious alternative is to use machines.

Machine Exercises:

All *leg press machines,* requiring either a seated or lying position, are suited to toe raises. All you have to do is press the weight to a straight leg position, rest the edge of the foot pedal on your toes, and extend your ankle joint. Unfortunately, this can be dangerous if the foot pedal slips off your toes; for this reason, they are *not* recommended. A host of professional gym equipment companies (all of which are small in comparison to Marcy, Nautilus, Paramount, or Universal) make specialized apparatuses for toe raises. Even though this is a popular exercise, the large equipment manufacturers don't make this kind of equipment.

A Final Word on Exercises

All equipment used in weight training, whether free weights or machines, is designed to afford you the wherewithall to develop your muscles. Most free weight exercises and most machines are designed to give you maximum effective isolation of the target muscle(s).

Some things never change, and the principle of isolation is one of them. But it won't take you more than a few visits to the gym to notice that a turn this way or a twist that way on any given exercise machine will yield slightly different results, or that an exercise designed to develop one muscle may be felt in a completely different location! For example, you'll feel squats more on your shoulders than in your legs. You may feel tricep push-downs more in your abdominals than in your triceps. Or, you'll get a burning sensation in your biceps when doing lat pull-downs.

Don't let this deter you from the exercise. When you do an exercise correctly, you'll feel it in the target muscle(s). That you also feel it elsewhere is incidental, and is the result of other muscles working to help the target muscle or stabilize a distant body part so the target muscle can work more efficiently. That is the nature of the human musculoskeletal system. There is nothing you can do about it. In fact, you shouldn't try: The added development received by these distant "helpers" and "stabilizers" will only add to your overall fitness and general body strength. Let it happen naturally.

Finally, don't be afraid to experiment with different movements, positions, and exercises! You'll find the ones that suit you best, and you'll have more fun in the process.

Sources

Manufacturers, Designers, and Photographers

MANUFACTURERS

Amerec
P.O. Box 3825
Bellevue, WA 98009
(206) 643-1000

AMF American
200 American Avenue
Jefferson, IA 50129
(515) 386-3125 (800) 247-3978

Avita
M & R Industries, Inc.
9215 151st Avenue N.E.
Redmond, WA 98052
(206) 885-1010

DP (Diversified Products)
309 Williamson Avenue
Opelika, AL 36802
(205) 749-9001

Elmer's Weights
P.O. Box 16326
Lubbock, TX 79490
(800) 858-4568

Fitness Products
Division of Quality Industries, Inc.
P.O. Box 254
Hillsdale, MI 49242
(517) 439-1581

Gravity Guidance, Inc.
1540 Flower Avenue
Duarte, CA 91010
(818) 303-4777

Huffy Sporting Goods
2018 First Street
Milwaukee, WI 53207
(414) 482-4240

KYGA
P.O. Box 24325
Denver, CO 80224
(303) 671-9347

Marcy Fitness Products
2801 West Mission Road
Alhambra, CA 91803
(818) 570-1222

McNeil Rebounder
P.O. Box 1110
Quincy, FL 32357
(800) 874-2900

Monark
Monark-Crescent AB
Varberg, Sweden 0340/86000

Nu-Barres
P.O. Box 3657
San Francisco, CA 94119
(415) 648-5230

Paramount Fitness Equipment Corporation
6450 East Bandini Blvd.
Los Angeles, CA 90040
(213) 721-2121

Pennypak
15 Linmoor Terrace
Lexington, MA 02173
(617) 863-1942

Precor USA
P.O. Box 1018
Redmond, WA 98073
(206) 881-8982

Space Weights
GraFar Corporation
7340 Fenkell
Detroit, MI 48238
(313) 862-9195

Stairmaster
Tri-Tech Inc.
Box 6708
Tulsa, OK 74156
(918) 425-5589

Tredex
Universal Fitness Products
20 Terminal Drive, South
Plainview, Long Island, NY 11803
(516) 349-8600

Triangle Health & Fitness Products
P.O. Box 30785
Raleigh, NC 27622
(919) 781-6256

Tunturi
P.O. Box 3825
Bellevue, WA 98009
(206) 643-1000

The West Bend Company
Dart Industries
West Bend, WI 53095
(414) 334-2311

DESIGNERS

David Bell, ASID
Donald Cotter
Design Multiples
225 Lafayette Street
New York, NY 10003
(212) 219-8430

Eric Bernard Designs
177 East 94th Street
New York, NY 10128
(212) 876-9295

Maurice Bernstein
435 East 57th Street
New York, NY 10022
(212) 759-2363

Samuel Botero Associates, Inc.
345 East 56th Street
New York, NY 10022
(212) 935-5155

Rus Calder
15 Park Avenue
New York, NY 10016
(212) 689-8166

Chris Chimera
294 West 11th Street
New York, NY 10014
(212) 924-0519

Denning and Fourcade Inc.
125 East 73rd Street
New York, NY 10021
(212) 759-1969

Rubén De Saavedra, ASID
225 East 57th Street
New York, NY 10022
(212) 759-2892

Carey Kirk
Interior Design
100 West 72nd Street
New York, NY 10023
(212) 206-1070

Richard D. Lawrence Associates
25 Sutton Place North
New York, NY 10022
(212) 752-2930

Robert Mihalik
Loft 96 Design
96 Prince Street
New York, NY 10012
(212) 431-8297

James Franklin Mitchell & Associates
172 Fifth Avenue
New York, NY 10010
(212) 620-7316

Michael Mostoller
456 Riverside Drive
New York, NY 10027
(212) 864-1998

Patino/Wolf Associates
400 East 52nd Street
New York, NY 10022
(212) 355-6581

David Snyder
Vice President, Fashion
Marshall Field
111 North State Street
Chicago, IL 60690
(312) 781-5741

Charles Swerz Associates
202 West 40th Street
New York, NY
(212) 921-7980

Walz Design Inc.
141 Fifth Avenue
New York, NY 10010
(212) 477-2211

PHOTOGRAPHERS

Peter Aaron
ESTO Photographics Inc.
222 Valley Place
Mamaroneck, NY 10543
(914) 698-4060

Hedrich-Blessing
11 West Illinois Street
Chicago, IL 60610
(312) 321-1151

Ralph Bogertman
34 West 28th Street
New York, NY 10001
(212) 889-8871

Derrick & Love Interior Photography
333 West 19th Street
New York, NY 10011
(212) 243-7339

Daniel Eifert
26 Second Avenue
New York, NY 10003
(212) 473-2562

Jon Elliott Photographer
329 West 85th Street
New York, NY 10024
(212) 799-8828

Phillip H. Ennis Photography
2935 Dahlia Avenue
Bladwin Harbor, NY 11510
(516) 379-4273

Norman McGrath Photography
164 West 79th Street
New York, NY 10024
(212) 799-6422

Peter Paige Photography
37 West Homestead Avenue
Palisades Park, NJ 07650
(201) 592-7889

Mark Ross Photography
345 East 80th Street
New York, NY 10021
(212) 744-7258

Ricardo Alberto Salas
126 Fifth Avenue
New York, NY 10011
(212) 929-6995

Index

Index

T

U

V

W

Y

Photo Credits

Paul Warchol © ESTO: 54–55

Roger Bester: 10, 13, 16, 19, 23, 25, 27, 29, 31, 33, 41, 98, 100, 102, 103, 105, 107, 109, 112, 113, 114, 115, 116, 118

Ralph Bogertman: 57 (left and right)

Derrick and Love: 72

Michael Dunne/EWA: 56, 58-59

Dan Eifert: 48-49, 49

Jon Elliott: 82,82-83

© Phillip H. Ennis: 60-61, 61, 62-63, 64-65, 68-69, 70 (inset), 70-71, 90-91, 92-93

Arthur Foti: 88, 89

Keith Glasgow: 111

Hedrich-Blessing: 86-87

Neil Lorimar/EWA: 80-81

Norman McGrath: 76-77

Don Morley: 94 (bottom)

Courtesy of Nike, Inc.: 30

Peter Paige: 66, 66-67, 73, 84-85, 85

Rex Features: 95 (left)

Mark Ross: 78, 78-79

Ricardo Alberto Salas: 50, 51

© Sipa-Press/Rex Features: 94 (top), 95 (right)

Jerry Tubby/EWA: 52, 53

Photo Trends/P. Kredenser/Shooting Star: 96 (right and left)

Photo Trends/ Steve Harvey/Shooting Star/ © Yoram Kahama: 97

Morley Von Sternberg/EWA: 74, 75

Model Photography by Roger Bester
Womens' Body Wear Provided Exclusively by Danskin
Other Accessories Provided Courtesy of Nike, Inc.

About the Authors

Philip Mazzurco is an editor and freelance writer. Author of THE MEDIA DESIGN BOOK (Macmillan, 1984), he is currently at work on BATH DESIGN (Whitney Library, 1986). Mazzurco is also a contributor to *Home Entertainment, Restaurant Design, Lighting Dimensions,* and *Playboy* magazines. He is a press member of the American Society of Interior Designers.

Frederick C. Hatfield, Ph.D., is a distinguished scholar as well as participant in the world of fitness. He is currently Editor-in-Chief of *Sports Fitness* magazine and has published widely in the health field. In addition to his academic interest in fitness, the author is the current World Champion in powerlifting and was a nationally ranked gymnast and Olympic-style weightlifter for several years.